JUDITH WILLS

ESCAPE THE

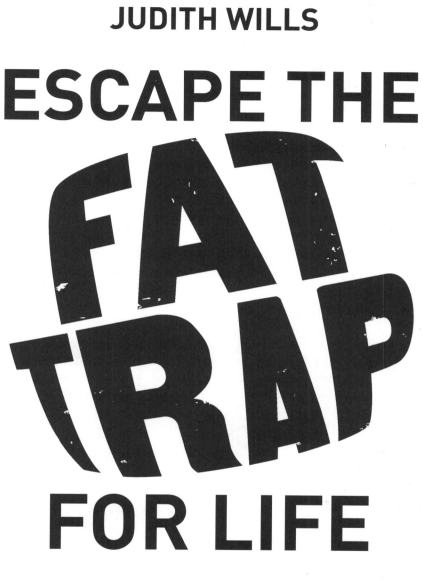

FAT
TRAP

FOR LIFE

Discover your body's natural intelligence and how to look good and feel better forever

D0542300

ARIES

Acknowledgements
The author would like to thank everyone who helped the book become reality, especially Kyle
and her brilliant team at Kyle Cathie. I_____ _____ ___ __ V___ O____ A___
Newman, Jane Turnbull, Lizzie Webb, R

Waltham Forest Libraries		
904 000 00206681		
Askews		23-Jul-2010
613.25		£9.99
2883004		B

First published in Great Britain in 2010
Kyle Cathie Limited
23, Howland Street
London W1T 4AY
general.enquiries@kyle-cathie.com
www.kylecathie.com

ISBN 978 1 85626 914 8

A Cataloguing in Publication record for this title is available from the British Library.

10 9 8 7 6 5 4 3 2 1

Judith Wills is hereby identified as the author of this work in accordance with Section 77
of the Copyright, Designs and Patents Act 1988.

All rights reserved. No reproduction, copy or transmission of this publication may be made
without written permission. No paragraph of this publication may be reproduced, copied
or transmitted save with written permission or in accordance with the provisions of the
Copyright Act 1956 (as amended). Any person who does any unauthorised act in relation
to this publication may be liable to criminal prosecution and civil claims for damages.

Text copyright © 2010 by Judith Wills
Design © 2010 by Kyle Cathie Limited

Design: Seagull Design
Editor: Vicky Orchard
Copy editor: Anne Newman

Printed and bound in Great Britain by Martins the Printers Ltd

Disclaimer
The advice in this book (and reporting of the advice from scientists across the world)
is intended for adults in normal health. If you have any specific health problems,
allergies etc. for which you are receiving medical advice, you should ask for more personal
recommendations about your diet – your own doctor can refer you to a dietician for
whatever help you need. The author and publisher cannot accept responsibility for illness
arising out of the failure to seek medical advice from a doctor.

Contents

Introduction

I confess. Twenty years ago, I used to write 'get slim quick' diet books, with names like *High Speed Slimming* and *A Flat Stomach in 15 Days*. And for all of the 1980s, as editor of a slimming magazine, I spent my days 'helping' people who couldn't lose weight, inventing new diets and angles to fill the pages and thinking up attention-grabbing cover lines.

A career in the media side of the diet industry wasn't something I'd planned. For several years, I had been a women's feature writer for various national magazines and newspapers, producing anything from celeb interviews to pieces on village schools about to close down. I was offered the job as editor of *Slimmer* magazine by chance, and at first, I turned it down, saying I found diets and the whole slimming business boring. But the managing editor felt that my scepticism might just give the magazine the edge it needed, and persuaded me I was the person to take charge. Reluctantly, I said I'd give it a go for six months. (I stayed for over ten years, until 1990, when my first diet book became a bestseller and I had a diet column signed and sealed with the *Daily Express*.)

While editing the magazine, I went with the flow, convincing myself that I was offering a service to the readers, helping them to achieve 'better' bodies, while providing myself with a reasonably lucrative career. But a small voice in my head was always there, quietly saying: 'Your heart's not really in this, is it?'

The truth is, while it was occasionally morale-boosting to help people (mostly women) lose weight and change their lives, I disliked much of what I had to do – accept advertising from dubious companies and assure readers that thin was the thing to be, and that they would all succeed in their slimming endeavours. Because I knew, that for over 90 per cent of readers, their diets would end in failure.

However, it was only when I made a promotional trip to Australia for my new diet paperback in the early '90s, and the media there dubbed me the 'Queen of Lean', that I realised I was promoting something I didn't really believe in. I found myself on live TV, protesting – much to the horror of the presenter

– that I wasn't the 'Queen of Lean' and that I believed, in fact, that people shouldn't be too thin.

When I returned to the UK, I made the decision to begin writing with a much more moderate, considered and long-term approach to the tricky subjects of weight, diets, food and health. I wanted to build a reputation as the voice of reason, when all around me seemed to want quick-fix diets and outlandish solutions to their body worries. In short, I wanted to tell the truth. I knew it would be a sure-fire way to reduce my income overnight from rather good to poor – or possibly non-existent – but it had to be done for my own conscience.

Thus, over the past twelve years or so, I have produced titles, some of which have sold well, but which were not designed to grab headlines. *The Food Bible*, *The Diet Bible*, *The Children's Food Bible* and *The Green Food Bible* were basically encyclopaedias, offering an unbiased look at their respective topics. At last, I was completely happy with the work I was producing and finally had peace of mind.

It was a government-sponsored seminar on obesity held at Whitehall in the spring of 2009 that made me decide to make one last return to the world of diets, scams, wild promises, myths, falsehoods and plain lies that so many of us live in today. I sat through the seminar for four hours and listened as MPs, forum leaders and various professionals from the fields of health, nutrition, obesity – the finest minds in their fields – talked, made promises and shared ideas (most of which I had heard ten, twenty, even thirty years earlier, and all of which had failed to bring about any change). Well, unless you count change in the form of rising obesity levels, diminishing activity levels and increases in eating disorders, of course.

I listened as food – one of my great pleasures – was discussed as if it were medicine or poison, the enemy or a recalcitrant child, depending on who was speaking. And I listened as the greatest health brains in the country talked about ways to persuade the population of the UK to keep their bodies active and fit – the unmistakeable underlying sentiment being that it was a 'battle' no one really believed they could win.

We spend huge amounts of time and energy on worrying and feeling guilty about the way we look, what we eat, whether we are too fat, too thin. We waste enormous amounts of time and money listening to everyone from bona fide doctors to bogus gurus, most of whom, when it comes down to it, know less about our bodies and the answers to our questions than we do ourselves. Yet, despite this, our bodies are collectively, steadily – and sometimes rapidly – becoming worse. Our efforts just aren't working.

On leaving the seminar, I knew that what was really needed was a book about the way things actually are for most of us today, rather than how they might be in an ideal world – one that identifies the problems and finds solutions. And I realised that the vital ingredient we all need in order to escape the fat trap is 'body IQ'.

IQ – intelligence quotient – is usually applied to our mental powers or, sometimes, to our emotional powers. But we rarely think of our physical IQ – knowledge and intelligence about our bodies, how they work naturally and what they need. The application of physical IQ (defined as 'the input of correct information, and the interpretation of that information') would empower every one of us to achieve the body we would like to – or perhaps, should – have. It would provide an escape from the fat trap (and, indeed, from the thin trap too).

Make no mistake – despite, or perhaps more accurately, because of, my background and disdain for sections of the 'diet industry' – I do think that your body is hugely important. The state it is in *does* matter – for your health, self-image, confidence and longevity. You shouldn't feel guilty about wanting to look good, lose weight (or gain it, if you need to) – but what you should do is to find out what is realistic, desirable and achievable without compromising yourself, your wallet or, ironically, your body.

This book will help you to do this in two key ways:

- It tells the truth about what really works, what really doesn't – and why.
- It tells you how to control and yet be kind to your body, thus satisfying its needs, as well as its wants, so that it may function properly and be the body you want to live inside.

As such, this is one of the best tools you will find to help you enjoy your life, your body, your food, to look and feel better and to escape the fat trap – for life.

Part One:
The Trap

1

The Tyranny of Skinny

- Each year over 10 million people in the UK and 40 million people in the USA begin a new diet; within five and a half weeks 50 per cent have given up, having wasted collectively, on average, £335 million (on products, gym memberships etc.) in the process.
- Of those who succeed in losing weight in the short term, 95 per cent have put all the weight back on within a year.
- It is estimated that over 80 per cent of adults in the UK have been on a diet at one time or another.
- Approximately 55 per cent of UK adults have bought products to help them lose weight – from pills to patches, miracle cures and detoxes (excluding books and videos).
- Eighty per cent of UK women and 45 per cent of men are unhappy with their appearance.
- In the UK and USA combined, approximately 12 million people suffer from eating disorders, such as anorexia.
- Twenty-six per cent of ten-year-old girls feel they aren't thin enough.
- It's been estimated that on average, women in the UK and USA spend ten years of their lives trying to be slimmer than they are, but end up fatter.

Most of us want to be thin, even if we pretend otherwise. Ask most women in the UK in their forties to sixties, and you'll find that they've spent most of their adult years fretting about whether they were thin enough.

But this is not a recent phenomenon. Many people cite the growth of the food industry after the Second World War as the beginnings of obesity and the need to diet. But read this:

'A new craze in women's fashion [has] burst upon the community. They call it "slimming". Many who practise it succeed in resembling famine victims – those who could become the most like living skeletons being the envy of their sisters.'

This was written about women – in one of the earliest diet books published in the UK – in 1926. While in 1929, a well-known theatrical impresario in London said of chorus girls: 'Many of them ruin their digestions by crazy dieting to keep slim.'

Research today, however, shows that men are almost as obsessed. The number of males on diets and/or getting body reshaping and retouching is rising steeply (for example, there has been an increase of over 50 per cent year on year in Botox for men and 200 per cent in two years for some types of cosmetic surgery), while the latest figures show that 25 per cent of people with eating disorders are now male.

And, horrifyingly, our children – even pre-school-aged children – are showing signs of being similarly body conscious. It doesn't help that dolls like Barbie and Bratz and cartoon females (such as Princess Tiana in *The Princess and the Frog*, whose waist is half the width of her head) are all size zero, without a doubt. And the Government's anti-obesity campaign, which includes allowing education authorities to weigh pupils and send warning letters to parents if a child is overweight, may actually be compounding this increasing childhood obsession with not being fat.

We obsess, we try, we fail, we try, we give up, we succeed, we revert. But in the long term, being thin, however much we want it and however hard we try, doesn't happen. The Catch 22 statistic is that two thirds of us are actually overweight or clinically obese. Which rather undermines the argument proposed by some that constantly seeing thin body images is a motivational tool which may help to prevent even more of us becoming even more overweight.

It is human nature to want what we can't have: when we're busy, we want more leisure time; when we're overrun with a hectic social life, we crave peace and solitude. And when our waists are bulging, we crave and admire slimness. We are at the opposite end of the scale from where we want to be, or *think* we want to be.

So let's take a look at this phenomenon, call it what you will – the 'tyranny of skinny', 'thin' or 'size zero syndrome' – more closely.

It is ironic that the female body was cleverly designed for carrying babies, giving birth and nurturing an infant, and yet women seem often to reject the body parts that are vital to this process – the breasts, the child-bearing hips, the extra fat. How strange that modern woman – the have-it-all person, the multi-tasker, the achiever, the intelligent, powerful being that she often is – can be reduced to a depressed bundle of neurosis if she has a blowout weekend and has put on three pounds by Monday morning.

But being comfortable with your figure is not necessarily connected with how you actually look, as numerous studies show. Most women think they look 'worse' (i.e. fatter or more out of proportion) than they really are. And having a 'good' figure doesn't necessarily guarantee you a good life. Just look at the celebrities whose bodies you most admire or crave and you will see the truth of that.

The Deception

The tyranny of skinny is a deception that works on different levels.

Firstly, there are the images of people you admire: TV personalities, film stars, models and so on. You see their photographs in magazines and on the net. They look slim, very slim. You know that many of these images are digitally altered, yet you look at them in awe and think that is how you too would look your best.

Secondly, there are the lies about what and how much they eat. Actress A says she eats like a horse and is just naturally thin. Model B says that she loves chocolate, but that she burns up lots of calories being on the go all day, and that explains her figure. The underlying message is that if these thin women can eat what they want and still stay thin, you must be eating *way* too much. This is damaging to your self-esteem and to the way you see yourself. Yet, most of these so-called role models are not telling the truth; they eat virtually nothing and many of them are exercise addicts too. Looking the way they do is neither easy nor fun – and it certainly isn't healthy. So don't let them make you think otherwise.

One of the UK's national daily newspapers has been running a series on what famous (slim) women eat in a week. While the average a woman should eat to maintain weight is around 2000 calories a day, every one of these women, *every one of them*, eats around a third less than that. They really watch what they eat – and by some standards, many of them would not be considered actually skinny at all, just slim.

Similarly, some keep quiet about the amount of exercise they do. Make no mistake, to get a body like Madonna's (should you want it) you would need to put in several hours a day of strenuous workouts – a level of exercise that could cause all kinds of physical and health problems for many of us.

And thirdly, there is the hype that increases your interest in crazy diets, as you read about the latest, greatest diet in almost any women's magazine, any week of the year. Well, you think – if it worked for her, I'll give it a try; she's rich, famous and slim and you don't get to be that way unless you're fairly bright and intelligent, so she must know what she's talking about. I'll give it a try.

But the fact is, as a recent USA overview of dieting methods reveals, a diet will work to lose you weight if it reduces your calorie intake. A crazy diet will do that. But a sensible, varied diet will do that too. All the crazy diet does is send YOU crazy after a week or even less, as it is not a normal way of eating. So then you stop, you put the pounds you lost back on and feel worse about yourself than you did at the start.

Still, it's hard to ignore the skinny messages. They may vary in their intent and in their delivery, but what they're all doing is asking you to jump on the bandwagon, implying that if you don't, you're somehow less of a person than you could be, or even that you're lazy (which could explain why a recent study found that being over average size greatly diminishes a woman's chance of landing a job at high management level). And on the flip side, they're suggesting that you too could look beautiful if you do jump on. Of course, it's hard to resist.

But who actually benefits from all this? It's not the skinny role models. Nor is it you. Let's have a closer look at where all the messages are really coming from. Who is the beneficiary? Because, believe me, they're all around – vultures, circling, waiting for you to succumb.

The Opposition – What You're Up Against

How did we get from admiring Marilyn and her fellow film stars of the 1950s to today – when Angelina, Cheryl, Agyness and beanpoles everywhere are held up as having bodies to die for? And some women do, literally. Die, that is.

I'll tell you how we got here.

The fashion and advertising industries

These have all kinds of ways of ensuring you only feel good when you're a size 10 (US 6) or below. In fact, in the industry, size 10 is more or less obese.

First, they choose beyond-thin models for the catwalk because these breastless girls show off the line of the clothes better, say the designers. This is partly true, but another important reason is that it is simply harder to design clothes when you have to take account of curves. Next, the press and PR offices of the designers (and the fashion stores) keep only small sizes of the clothes in stock, so the models used by the photographers have to be thin to fit into them. Thus, you'll see only photos of ultra-slim girls modelling the clothes you are supposed to covet. So, you assume that's how women ought to look.

Now, because the models at most of the agencies are thin (because they have to be), when an advertising agency wants to book a model they have no choice but to go with thin too. So the 'ideal' is reinforced, yet again.

And that's just one of the reasons why we get anorexia worship, with internet sites devoted to promoting the disease and idolising women so thin they are on the point of starvation.

Finally, this is compounded by the shops themselves. While there are exceptions, if you want to treat yourself to a designer outfit for a wedding or a holiday or just because you're worth it – woe betide you if you're over a size 12. You won't find the stock. This is in part because again the designers don't want to see their exclusive designs on women with anything less than stick-thin, perfect bodies.

It is also, in part, down to the high-street chains. Mass-market clothes are produced in a factory and cannot take account of the huge variations in shape and size in any population. Thus, it is in their interests, too, to try to get us to conform to a few sizes. If they only have to produce sizes 10, 12 and 14 for example in one style, they will make more money than if they have to produce it in sizes 8–22. It's easier, quicker and, therefore, cheaper for them to get us to do the hard work. (And guess what – the smaller you are, the less material your clothes will use, so they save on costs that way too!)

FASHION'S IDEA OF FAT

During 2009, I read several laughable pieces in the papers written by journalists attached to the fashion industry, claiming that curves were at last 'in' on the catwalk, and also trying to sound as if everyone were delighted about this. 'The backlash against size zero!' they trumpeted.

This is all well and good, until you realise that the industry's idea of curvy is a non-funny joke. For example, the latest 'discovery' – a Dutch model called Lara Stone – has been described as 'a world away from skinny', 'a real woman with curves', 'an inclusive body shape' (meaning you and I should think of her as one of us ordinary people).

The model herself is not that happy with her size, and is quoted as saying, 'If you're confronted with colleagues half your size, you think, "F***, I'm really fat!"'

Now, hear this: Lara Stone is a *huge* size 8 (USA 4).

Fashion and beauty journalists

I used to be a beauty editor – it was my first job as a writer and I did it for two long, boring years. Even then, at the tender age of twenty, I realised that both cosmetics and fashion were in part a con designed to extract money from impressionable young women. And it was the job of the writers on the magazines (which relied heavily on advertising revenue) to make people feel bad about themselves unless they did/bought X, Y or Z.

In those days, beauty and health were usually covered by the same journalist, certainly on the women's magazines, and diet, size and weight were part of the 'health' remit. They wrote to encourage readers to get slim enough to wear the latest fashions, as if they were not just options, but completely vital for readers' credibility and attractiveness. And, in the next feature, they wrote to persuade readers they were fat enough to need the latest beauty treatments and slimming foods and supplements. That was the route to approbation from the fashion, cosmetic and pharmaceutical companies who were the mainstay advertisers for the fashion magazines, and thus to approval from the editor. Everybody knew that if the illusion wasn't maintained, there would be no advertising, no magazine, no job.

Sadly, thirty-plus years later, writers are still peddling the same messages. And it's not just those on the young women's glossies and celeb magazines. This is a passage I read in 2009 in *The Times* newspaper, written by one of their leading columnists:

'It was only a matter of time before the bare tummy returned, but if there is a part of the female form we collectively want to hide, it's the expanse between our breasts and our hipbones. Unfortunately, trends wait for no one's insecurities, so you're going to have to suck it up and suck it in.'

The piece went on to describe various 'solutions' to the bare-tummy problem (the cheapest of which cost £20).

And again in *The Times*, a writer put panic into every reader over a size 10 and with a hint of flab or cellulite, when discussing bikini-worthy bodies: 'Last year, passing the bikini challenge was desirable, now it's a matter of survival. It separates the "got-its" from the "not-quites". It's now a requirement of women who want to stay visible.'

Even Oprah Winfrey, America's queen of TV, with her own big-circulation magazine, *O* (mantra – to promote personal growth), while setting a good example by not being too skinny herself, spends her time obsessing in public about her inability to stabilise her weight, and apparently allowed the stick-thin Editor of US *Vogue*, Anna Wintour, to persuade her to lose weight before she could appear on the magazine's cover.

And there are hundreds more examples I could quote you. Once you begin to notice these insidious pleas to become skin and bone and/or spend money in doing so, you won't stop seeing them. But that's good – the more you see, the more you may recognise the truth and the motivation behind their message.

The digital age

Ubiquitous digital retouching of photos before they are published ensures that tiny hints of flab are photoshopped out, waists are thinned and legs are shaped or slimmed, so that any model who had the temerity to be anything other than 'perfect', and/or perfectly thin, is so once on the page. Of course, while many of us now understand that this is what happens, I am quite sure that there are plenty of young girls, young women (and many older ones too) who still can't help themselves from feeling bad about their own ordinary size 12 or 14 or 16.

Even fifteen years ago, when I appeared on the cover of some of my own diet books, and at the time had quite a 'good' figure at a reasonably toned size 12, each and every image was airbrushed to make me look better. I still look at the cover of *Size 12 in 21 Days* and cringe because I hate what they did to my body and my face. On another occasion, I appeared sitting sideways on a bar stool in the colour supplement of a tabloid Sunday newspaper, and they carved out my belly area so much I looked literally deformed, at least in my eyes. It was around that time that I began to realise that I wanted out.

The leisure and fitness industry

Swish gyms and spas can be daunting places to try to get fit if you're flabby, overweight – and with the often-accompanying fragile self-esteem.

The changing rooms and workstations are awash with beautiful people sporting not a spare ounce of flesh and to an insecure size 16 or over this can send out similar messages to those you're getting from fashion and media – 'Don't stop till you look like THIS!'

If you decide never to return, this may not be a wholly bad thing – I believe there are better places and ways to get fitter – and for more on that read Chapter Eight.

There is also a danger of getting completely sucked in to the fitness and gym ethic, so that – like 1 per cent of people in the UK and USA – you find exercise has become your fix, your addicton. Like anorexics or alcoholics, sufferers often need therapy to overcome their obsession and begin living again and, indeed, exercise addiction is linked in many cases with eating disorders and the compulsion to become thin.

The moralists

Gluttony – the over-consumption of anything, but usually taken to mean food – was one of the seven deadly sins in the Christian religion. Another was sloth – laziness. There are still people around today who may make some of us feel that we are somehow immoral for being rounded, eating well, looking a little large. My own mother felt that way, though she disguised it well most of the time. I still remember the day I sat with her, a few years before she died, a tiny, bird-like creature who ate like a bird, too, and for many years had abhorred waste and excess and admired thrift and energy. She was talking about a neighbour. 'I don't like her coming in here,' she said. 'She's fat. I don't like fat people.'

I know she always preferred me when I was slimmer rather than, say, after a baby or a period of ill health a few years back when I had put on some weight. If I wore something 'slimming' when I visited her, she would always exclaim with delight, 'Oooh – you've lost weight!' She couldn't help it – she simply had that mindset. But the underlying implication was that thin is good, fat is bad, and this is something that creeps into many normal, loving relationships, almost, but not quite, unnoticed.

Diet product, companies and clinics

You know, obviously, that an advertisement is selling you something, and these days many of us do think twice before believing what we're told in the ads or being taken in by what is implied in a photograph or image. Which is why indirect selling through promotion, PR and clever marketing is a much better way to get you hooked.

PR, marketing and ad agencies place products with celebs and get them to plug them. From books to pills to remedies to gyms, spas, weight-loss programmes, patches – celebs sell it all. And they're paid to do it.

Similarly, cosmetic surgeons often give celebs free tucks, lifts, reductions and so on in return for their 'pro' stance on the cosmetic surgery industry. And, in turn, their positive take makes you think that invasive surgery may not be such a nasty, dangerous procedure, after all.

And think of all the spas, clinics, health farms, treatment centres, clubs and more – all there to help you achieve your thin goal. If you suddenly decided your money would be better spent on a nice bottle of wine and a beach holiday they'd rapidly go out of business.

Television and film

Firstly, a common lament heard by actors of both sexes, presenters and anyone who appears on TV and film is that it is almost a given that they need to be slim (and young, but that's another story). If anyone who is overweight has the audacity to appear on TV, it is either because they are amazingly funny, incredibly pushy and confident or taking part in a get-slim series. This was perfectly demonstrated when the singer Susan Boyle appeared on the TV show *Britain's Got Talent* in 2009, and her appearance caused a national outcry – not only did she have unfashionably cut, greying hair and wore no make-up – but she was *at least* a size 14! Unforgivable! Within weeks she had been 'made over'. Our screens have a lot to answer for.

TV also has to take some of the blame for why our celebs think they need to be so thin. It is quite true that on screen, bodies look fatter than they really are. And with wide screen this effect is even worse – if you stand at the edge of a group of people on TV, you will look twice as wide as you really are. So many people who appear on TV are quite paranoid about their weight, and will go to great lengths to keep themselves slightly underweight to cancel out the unfair screen effect.

Mass market media

Even the middle- and so-called up-market press will often concentrate on a woman's appearance, rather than what she does, says or is. For example, France's first lady, Carla Bruni, who speaks several languages, fights for women's rights across the world, sets classical poetry to music and has bestselling albums, was made fun of in the *Daily Telegraph* for not looking as fashionable/sexy as Spain's first lady when they were pictured together, while the middle-market papers openly compared her (apparently, inferior) bottom to that of her rival.

But it is the down-market tabloids, internet sites aimed at women and celeb watchers and the weekly celeb magazines who are the main culprits in picking over all kinds and shapes and sizes of celebs and sneering at the slightly larger ones, while praising those who manage to remain a size zero. But just to prove they've got our best interests at heart, really, they will throw in the occasional 'shock, horror' comment about someone who has gone just a tad too far with her starvation diet and is growing body hair.

Such is the influence of these commentaries, that it isn't just us, the punters, who are moved to try to diet. Even the people who are dissected in the columns and have their curves pointed out in red arrows on their photos, aren't immune. For example, one woman with a previously healthy, beautiful body – one so admired that she was a lingerie model – Kelly Brook, found herself compelled to go on a crash diet after seeing a paparazzi photo of herself in one of the celeb mags.

As these forms of media have become our new best friends, they have also taken over the role of best friend. We listen to what they say and, often, we take their advice and want to please them. But, as Gwyneth Paltrow would say, really, they are the 'frenemy' (an enemy posing as a friend).

Next time you buy a celeb mag, look for the pages (and there are always a few) where the paparazzi have spotted some previously admired B-lister who is now looking less than perfect: a bit of cellulite on the thighs; a pair of fat knees, suddenly exposed by a short skirt or bit of breeze; a double chin or a man boob; even a few spots. While being intrusive and, no doubt, making the celebs in question less than happy, these pictures prove that it *is* all an illusion. Take away the good lighting, the clothes, the fake tan, the re-touching, the digital slimming, the impossible diet, and the truth is there for us all to see.

Put simply, bodies are imperfect. Perfect does not exist.

The 'ideal' body

Who was it who first decided what the ideal body looks like? Well there has been a lot of research on what the 'average' bust, waist and hips is, based on population studies. But, of course, as we get larger and larger (which we are doing) then the average goes up too. So if the 'average' 36–26–36 figure of the 1950s was the ideal body then, the average 39–32–41 body should be the ideal now. But it isn't. We still want the 1950s body as a maximum, and smaller, if possible.

I cut out thirty photos from the papers of the skinniest catwalk models, wearing the skimpiest outfits I could find (so their bodies were properly on display) and took them around a dozen or so acquaintances of all ages and sizes and both sexes and asked them for an opinion.

Every one of them – male and female alike – disliked them. The women said they did not want to look like that, and the males weren't attracted to them. Why? Far too thin. They were described by more than one person as 'a freak show'.

I also showed them the latest copy of the Figleaves lingerie brochure, in which the models are all nicely curvaceous, with what I would call average to slim, but not thin, bodies. Both the men and women liked these images.

This proved what I had suspected – that while underweight women may look OK with their clothes on, 'normal' women actually have more going for them with their clothes off. Maybe they have more fun with sex, better sex.

So there is hope. But even if we recognise that we don't want to be quite that thin, if we see the models regularly – which we do – the catwalk distorts our view of what a woman looks like. Modern models are the reason why it is often said today that Marilyn Monroe – one of the most-envied women of the twentieth century for her looks and figure – was fat. Put a photo of her beside one of a catwalk skeleton, or even a Victoria Beckham or a Kate Moss, and she will look fat. But according to journalist Sara Buys, who had the chance in 2009 to try on the actual skin-tight red dress that Marilyn wore in *Gentlemen Prefer Blondes*, and was photographed wearing it, Marilyn was not a size 16 – she had a natural 91cm (36in) bust (which always looked bigger because of her narrow back), a 58cm (23in) waist and 89cm (35in) hips. That is the truth. Even at her largest, Sara estimated, Marilyn would have been no more than a size 12.

It made me laugh when I read a recent wave of articles in the Sunday supplements, written by the fashion journalists, about how since the global recession, we all – the fashion industry included – are 'celebrating the fuller figure'. A handful of people may be doing that, but a flick through the pages of all the papers reveals that nothing, but nothing, has actually changed.

From my own research, if you put both sexes' preferences together you get something like the 'perfect' blueprint, the image that dominates women's thoughts and meets their goal:

- Even face with big eyes, small nose, large lips, firm jaw
- Strong shoulders, straight back, medium to large breasts, narrow, preferably long, waist (longer than average gap between lower ribcage and hips)
- Slim, but toned arms
- Small to medium hips and medium bottom, slightly rounded, but very firm and high
- Slim, but shapely legs, non-bony knees, slim ankles, pretty feet

I do know a few women who conform to most of this must-have list, but the majority of them have been surgically enhanced, so that doesn't count. (More about that later, see p. 140.)

Whether you want to be like a catwalk model, a page-three girl, a singer, actress or TV presenter, the fact is that you're always comparing yourself – your body – with someone else, and you're always finding yourself, and your body, wanting. This is all fodder for the fat trap from which you are trying to escape.

Until these so-called skinny or slim/perfect role models change – which is unlikely to happen in the foreseeable future – then the only way to sanity and body intelligence for ourselves, is to change our own attitudes; to try to kill the body envy and the gullibility in believing that being a size zero – or even, for most of us, a size 8 – is a natural phenomenon and that you can get there and stay there while eating normally. You can't.

How to Say Goodbye to All That, Gladly

You thought you were making your own decisions. Now you know you are probably not. That should make it a whole lot easier to make different decisions based on what's good and right for you, rather than for someone who has your best interests at the very bottom of their list – or, let's be honest, not on their list at all.

So let's now have a look at some of the reasons why skinny may not be what you want after all.

The link between thinness and physical ill health

What is thinness? Well, in adults, it is officially deemed to be a body mass index (BMI) which falls below 18.5, while a 'normal' healthy weight is anything between 18.5 and 25. While there are professionals who disagree with the concept of BMI as a way to measure under-, normal or overweight, it is currently the only internationally accepted and 99 per cent reliable formula we have, so I use it here. It is a better measure of thinness, in fact, than it is of overweight, a subject I will return to in Chapters Two and Three.

So let's have a look at a couple of examples.

You are 1.7m (5ft 7in) and you weigh 54kg (8½ stone). To calculate your BMI, you divide your weight in kilograms by your height in metres squared (54 ÷ (1.7 x 1.7) 2.89 = 18). Thus, your BMI is 18.7 and you are clinically underweight.

Most models and a high percentage of 'celebrities' are slimmer than this. Model and Miss Universe contestant Stephanie Naumoska, for example, is 1.8m (5ft 11in) and weighs 48kg (7 stone 8lb). Her BMI is, therefore, 14.9.

FACT

Around the same time Marilyn Monroe was queen of the movies, a slimmer, taller model (albeit with a large bust) came along and became just as famous. Her name was Barbie – Barbie doll. She's fifty years old now and still as impossibly slim as ever, while the women who were first bought Barbies back in 1959 still struggle. No wonder even young girls want to diet.

Low body weight is linked with the following health problems:

- Cessation of menstrual periods and infertility.
- Increased risk of osteoporosis (bone mineral depletion and loss of bone mass).
- Risk of malnutrition (e.g. shortfall of vitamins and minerals for general good health and body maintenance).
- High risk of inadequate protein intake for lean tissue (muscle) replacement and maintenance (it is not just your obvious 'muscles' which are lean tissue; the heart and other organs are composed of lean tissue too, meaning if you maintain underweight for periods of time, you may weaken your heart and organs and put yourself at risk of organ failure).
- High risk of inadequate essential fat intake which can result in dry skin, impaired brain function and a loss of all the health protection benefits these fats offer (for example, protection from heart disease, some cancers, immune deficiency diseases, arthritis and Alzheimer's).
- Diminished immune system, meaning you are more likely to suffer from bacterial and viral infections and take longer to recover.

FACT
Body fat is not a sin – in women, a reasonable amount of body fat is an advantage. It helps to insulate our bodies and protect our bones; it produces the hormone leptin which boosts the immune system and can help enhance our mood; it is vital for fertility and reproduction and vital both during and after the menopause to help boost oestrogen hormone activity and to protect against osteoporosis.

The link between thinness and mental health

While not all thin people suffer from an eating disorder, as such (i.e. one which has been clinically diagnosed), and there are, of course, some thin, healthy people who do eat reasonable amounts or even a lot, among certain populations (teenagers, young adults, mid-life women are particularly prone) extreme thinness is linked with anorexia (the avoidance of food/calories/ particular types of food to maintain extremely low body weight, sometimes coupled with over-exercising), bulimia (vomiting after eating on a regular basis to avoid absorption of calories/fat/carbohydrates) and/or exercise addiction.

All these conditions have been linked with body-image problems. The sufferer frequently has a false picture of how she or he looks, believing themselves to be overweight. The condition may be triggered by problematic life events at home, college or work.

And, while a genetic element has been found in cases of anorexia (some experts believe certain people are born with a predisposition to develop the condition), a high percentage of anorexics and bulimics have been found to have problems such as low self-esteem.

Whether it's the psychological issues that trigger the eating disorders, or vice versa, is a conundrum which continues to be analysed and debated among health professionals, but one fact emerges strongly – that the process of becoming and remaining stick-thin when that isn't your natural body weight or shape does not make you happy.

But you don't need to be anorexic for the thin dream to give you psychological problems. And, worryingly, women with daughters may pass their own body anxieties on – girls as young as five read and absorb messages from their mothers about dieting, the 'importance' of being thin and counting calories.

The link between *trying* to be thin and mental health

Even if you don't get there, and you don't achieve the size, the weight, the perfection for which you strive, the process of trying to get there is just as damaging.

FACT
- Eighty-three per cent of young college women spend much of their time dieting, no matter what they weigh, according to a survey published in *Nutrition Journal* in the US, while 45 per cent of American women are on a diet on any given day. And the numbers of men doing the same thing grows every year, with 25 per cent of males on a diet on any given day.
- By their teens, over half of girls practise unhealthy diet-related behaviour, such as skipping meals, fasting or taking laxatives according to a US report in 2005.
- A 2006 magazine survey of young women found that one in three thought about their body shape most of the time every day. This was not in a positive way but negatively, reducing their self-confidence, reinforcing their poor body image. Indeed, over half said their body image spoiled their sex lives.
- Each time a woman or man embarks on a new diet to try to lose weight, and fails, or loses then regains the lost weight, this also reduces self-confidence and reinforces poor body image.

The Tyranny of Skinny: Are You At Risk?

Here are five key points to show when/whether you're at risk from becoming (or are already) a victim of the tyranny of skinny, followed by some simple suggestions for how to change your behaviour and/or thought patterns in order to escape:

1. *You weigh yourself daily – perhaps even more often. You even check your weight on other people's scales when you get the chance.*
   Compulsive weighing shows obsessive body-image problems and an irrational belief that measurable weight loss can take place in hours rather than over a realistic period of time. (In fact, short-term weight loss can only be comprised of body fluids, rather than fat.)
   If you're a hyper scale-hopper you should, at least in the short term, throw out the scales, rely only on looser feel of waistbands for a sense of weight loss, and concentrate on how you feel (e.g. more alert, less breathless, more stamina), rather than how you look or what you weigh.

2. *You avoid a long list of behaviours or circumstances (e.g. buying new clothes or applying for a new job, ditching the dead-end boyfriend) and tell yourself you will allow these to happen once you are at what you consider a suitable weight.*
   The belief that your life is 'on hold' until you lose weight, and that overweight is intimately linked with what you are allowed to do in terms of success, goals, experiences, is a dangerous, but extremely common one.
   Yet research shows that those people who are most successful in reaching and/or maintaining a healthy weight are those who enjoy their lives with an outgoing, positive attitude, and that self-esteem is a major factor in the ability to find contentment with a realistic body shape.

3. *You constantly compare your own body with other people's – in the streets, in changing rooms, at work, at nightclubs. You feel happy if you see larger people, who make you feel better – but if you're surrounded by smaller people, your confidence plummets.*
   Frequent comparisons like this mean that you're spending a lot of your time on creating negative thoughts about other people and

not enough time on more worthwhile interactions, such as sharing ideas, thoughts and feelings with the people you meet.

In body-image tests, it has been found that women typically believe themselves to look larger than they really are in comparison with others. Time spent in places and in activities which don't focus on how people look will help to diminish the negative-comparison syndrome, or at least to make it less important. Sometimes talking to the people whose bodies you feel are better than yours can help too – you may discover that they also have a poor body image; they may even have been envying your own size and shape.

4. *You choose your friends by their size and their ability to make you feel better about yourself, rather than for other attributes.*
   We've all heard about women who choose fat friends to boost their own chances with men, or simply to make themselves look thinner. It's not a cliché – it is true of more women than you might imagine (and I say women because men seem less inclined to use this trick) and it is a classic symptom of being under the skinny thumb.

   If this sounds like you, make a conscious effort to keep your larger friend. If she ever decides to lose a few pounds for health reasons, encourage her. This will boost your own confidence by reinforcing the belief that you are actually a good friend, rather than a selfish one. The truth is that women of any size who don't go out worrying what strangers are thinking about their looks are more likely to be positive, relaxed, fun and enjoying life. This can be true whether you are slim, average or overweight.

5. *Your wardrobe is full of clothes that are too small for you – clothes that you've bought thinking you'll soon be slim enough to wear them.*
   Every time you open your wardrobe you are reminded of the fact that you think you are overweight, and you don't like being that size. Your self-esteem plummets and another day begins with the choice of an old tried-and-tested outfit or a day wearing something that is too tight.

   Give the clothes that are too small to charity. That will make you feel good. If you can't afford a new wardrobe, buy some clothes in the right size from the same charity shop. That will reinforce the feeling that – if you need to – you may still lose weight, but in the meantime you have some things to wear that didn't cost too much.

If, by the time you have finished reading this book, you decide you are happy with your weight and shape, you can send those back to the charity shop and treat yourself to some new clothes in your size!

These five 'at risk' signals are just a few examples of how we behave when we're being controlled by the tyranny of skinny. There are more. Think about how you behave and the negative influences the skinny ideal has on your life.

In conclusion, being thin, wanting to be thinner, feeling fat, being fat, wanting to be thinner – it's all part of the same problem – a collective body obsession; the deep-rooted anxiety about looks that fills more time for many of us than worrying about our work, our family or anything else.

One reason for the obsession is because many of us just don't know for sure how we should look; how we want to look, even. One friend says that we're perfect as we are at size 14, another friend pulls us aside and tells us to 'get some self-respect, lose a stone'. And then we read that what men actually like is not skin and bones, but flesh and fat.

No wonder being average, a healthy 'normal' size is so hard to achieve – we don't know what it is.

So let me say this: you probably aren't on TV or a catwalk model. You are in real life. What people see is what you are. You have no need to conform to an ideal (yours or anyone else's).

There are, in fact, several health advantages to being female and slightly plump (with a BMI at the high range of 'normal'). But if you're naturally skinny, if you're eating well and feel healthy, you're probably fine, too.

What makes life interesting, anyway, is not our sameness but our differences. What you want to be is yourself, but the best you can be, in terms of health and a healthy shape and size.

You need to embrace each and every part of you – everything that makes you unique, every bit of you that you can't change; then you can consider the rest and come to reasonable conclusions about what could alter, why and how. And that's where body IQ comes in.

But first, we need to look at the other side of the coin – obesity – and its place in the fat trap ...

2

The Tyranny of Fat

Having presented in Chapter One a picture of the many forces conspiring to make people go to ridiculous lengths to be skinny at any cost, I make no apology for now turning to the opposite end of the spectrum – obesity.

- There are 400 million adults worldwide who are obese and 1.6 billion who are overweight.
- Approximately 70 per cent of adults in the UK and USA are overweight or obese.
- It is estimated that by 2030, 87 per cent of all women will be overweight.

There are now more overweight than under- or normal-weight people in the world – and that figure includes famine-hit and poverty-stricken countries. How did we get to be so large, and just why are so many of us, in so many parts of the world, under the thumb of surplus weight we can't shift? The reasons for obesity are both many and complex ... or few and simple, depending on which way you look at the issue. One thing is for certain though: lots of circumstances, thoughts and people, individuals, organisations and huge multi-national companies – each with their own agenda – are contributing to the obesity epidemic.

To clarify the undoubted weight of the problem we need to go back to its beginnings.

A Short History of Human Weight

Hunter-gatherers were not fat. Although I cannot prove it, I feel reasonably confident in making this statement. Before the advent of farming, around 12,000 years ago, when man – and woman – learnt how to sow seeds, and later how to domesticate animals for food, meaning they had to have a 'fixed abode', the accumulation of body fat would not just have been hard – it would have been almost impossible.

The two irrefutable factors involved in weight gain are simple: an abundance of food and paucity of activity. For early man, neither of these was an option. To find enough food to live on, the early tribes would have needed to hunt long and hard – for nuts, seeds, leaves, fruits, wild animals, fish – thus neatly burning the calories in what they did eat well before it had a chance to settle and force them to loosen their loin cloths. And without the convenience of central heating and thermal underwear, they would also have used up extra energy in the quest to keep warm – shivering does burn calories.

This is why historically, in some parts of the world, body fat was prized. It signified affluence – that you had access to plenty of food without physical toil. Indeed, today, families suffering famine across the world may look at someone with a fat layer with envy, and rightly so.

But beginning gradually in the Western world in the mid- to late nineteenth century, then more rapidly over the decades that followed, that prized layer of body fat evolved from being the privilege of the rich, to the right – and then the curse – of the millions. Food became readily available, then abundant, then over-abundant (at least in some of the countries of the world).

The natural order of things was lost. For example, the spring season every year used to be a time of natural cutting back of calories (as the foods harvested in autumn and stored for the winter had mostly gone, and the first of the new season's crops would not be harvested until early summer).

When it was all but too late to see what we had done, we found that we still wanted the food, but not the surplus body fat that came with it. But by that time, we had almost completely lost the ability to abstain. More importantly, we had lost the lifestyle and the instincts that helped early man to use energy – to recognise balance naturally (or unconsciously): the equation between food intake and calorie-burning that once, for thousands of years, kept us slim and fit.

So it isn't our fault if we are fat. It truly isn't. But it is still possible to alter our behaviour and thought patterns and get ourselves out of the fat trap. By reconnecting with our long-lost body intelligence, while avoiding the tyranny of skinny, we can regain some much-needed balance.

But before we move on, I'd like to offer you some guidelines to help you decide just how dominated – or otherwise – you are by the tyranny of fat. Look at the key points and see how many of them you identify with.
If you can recognise yourself in even three or four of them, your life may well be dominated by feeling, or being, overweight.

The Tyranny of Fat: Are You At Risk?

Here are ten key points to show when/whether your life is being ruled by the tyranny of fat:

1. *You make sure your fridge, freezer and larder are always well stocked, and when you leave home, even for a short while, you take a bag filled with snack foods. You feel uneasy, or even panicked, when you are 'trapped' anywhere (e.g. a bus, lecture room) without immediate access to food.*

   This behaviour is a throwback to hunter-gatherer man, when people needed to eat their fill because they were never sure where the next meal was coming from. The supermarkets have cashed in on this instinct and encourage us to think this way, even though we all know, really, that the food isn't going to disappear from the shops overnight, even if that meteor does hit the earth.

   Many of us haven't relearnt our behaviour, so we still stock up when the going is good, 'just in case' of famine or disaster. We no longer understand that experiencing occasional mild pangs of hunger doesn't mean we are about to die from malnutrition. The modern habit of grazing on snack foods, such as chocolate, crisps and cookies rather than, as in our recent past history, eating once or twice a day, or, as in our more distant history, when man would snack, but on low-calorie or metabolism-boosting items, such as fresh fruits or nuts from the trees, means that we have an assured and steady supply of food to hand. Without this supply, slim people tend not to fret, while overweight and obese people do.

2. *You avoid opportunities to be physically active. You prefer to spend time in front of the computer or TV to taking a walk. It's a long time since you rode a bike or a horse or participated in sport – watching it with a box of chocs is much more your sort of thing. You drive everywhere; your hobbies are all passive and you feel that your size, in any case, precludes you from taking much exercise.*

   While it is possible to be slim and also an unfit non-exerciser (and indeed large numbers of people do belong in that category), obesity and the sedentary lifestyle go hand in hand. And it's a downward spiral – the fatter you get, the less activity you do and the more your health suffers. Demoralisation sets in and you simply give up.

3. *You plan your days around mealtimes, and if a decision between friends/food, work/food or intellectual/social life/food has to be made, the food nearly always wins. For example, you pass on the chance to attend a seminar on a topic you're very interested in because you would miss your lunch; or you turn down an invitation to dinner with a friend you haven't seen in a while because she's vegetarian or can't cook; you choose your holidays based on the quality/quantity of the food you will receive (e.g. an all-inclusive hotel or cruise), rather than for the scenery, weather or architecture.* This shows that your priority is food. It is more important to you than anything else. This means that your world, with all its possibilities, and your potential to live a fulfilled and meaningful life are narrowed and restricted. You may also experience guilt (because you realise what is happening), anger, and even self-loathing because of your inability to escape from the control food exerts over you.

4. *You always buy and prepare more food than you think will be needed. Faced with the choice of a medium or a large food item, you will most often go for the larger one, even though logic tells you that the smaller one is plenty for however many people you need to feed. At home, whether cooking for yourself or others, you will 'make extra' – the bigger casserole, the larger pie, the extra handful of spaghetti – as in your mind there is nothing worse than people not having enough to fill their bellies. And you're not making double so that you can do the green thing and freeze a meal – you're making more so people can eat more.* Most people do this today. It's a different version of key point no. 1 above – erring on the side of generosity, just in case.

5. *You use food/drink as a reward – after exercise, a tricky meeting or conversation or on completion of a task, for example. You express your relief or reward yourself through a 'treat', such as chocolate, biscuits or wine.*
This is often a throwback to childhood when Mum or Dad would do the same for you: 'If you do your homework/eat your greens/sit quietly, you can have some sweets/ice cream/cake.' It is a hard habit to break – but it can be done.

6. *You use food as a crutch – when you are lonely, bored, worried, depressed, tired, stressed. This is known as 'comfort eating'. A study*

conducted by the Mental Health Foundation found that more Britons than ever before are living with anxiety-related disorders and so, hardly surprisingly, it has also been found that we are eating more of the old-fashioned 'comfort' foods, such as treacle tart and steamed puddings.

Comfort eating is so widespread that I believe most of us do it at least sometimes. When life gets tough food (or drink) is one of the easiest things to turn to – it doesn't answer back and provides instant pleasure. And because the foods associated with 'treats', such as carbohydrates, desserts, chocolate have become so overabundant, since food manufacturers cottoned on back in the 1960s that these items are some of the cheapest to produce and the easiest to get us to eat (through advertising), they are the ones we most tend to get 'hooked' on. However, comfort eating quickly turns sour for most people as it is followed by guilt and, almost inevitably, weight gain. Some comfort.

7. *You avoid situations that may draw attention to or disapproval of your weight. So you don't go on holidays that involve stripping down to a swimsuit or shorts and T-shirt.*

   This is another life-diminishing consequence of overweight. Feeling fat means you feel you are judged by everyone who looks at you (with the possible exception of other fat people who, ironically, may often have their own agenda for wanting to keep *you* fat). Feeling fat makes you want to achieve the opposite effect of what you feel your body is doing – you want to be invisible.

   Lack of self-confidence is much more common in overweight people than it is in underweight or normal-weight-range people. Being fat/obese is often a lonely road to travel (surprisingly, as so many of us are overweight, we still feel it is our problem, not a shared problem with a shared solution). Other people's disapproval also increases the sense that any attempt at losing weight will be hopeless.

   These feelings often manifest themselves in withdrawal and depression, or, less often, in being a people pleaser (see no. 10, below).

8. *You avoid situations that may trigger your own negative feelings about your size. For example, you don't apply for a promotion at work that you know you deserve and are capable of, either because you feel*

*your size may prevent you from doing your best at the interview, or
because you think the interviewer may believe that you must lack
self-discipline because you are fat.*

Putting life on hold until you are slim is a very common mindset. It
stems from a lack of confidence in your own abilities or capabilities
and the belief that you are unattractive to others and will not be
a 'proper person' until you lose weight. And this is not just
paranoia. It is a fact, in many areas of life, that fat people are
discriminated against – in the job market (particularly for women),
in relationships and in education.

9. *Much of your 'thinking time' – when you're travelling, in bed, in the
   bath, for example – is spent obsessing about the way you look, and
   thinking about what you'd like to do when you are slim (which you
   will be one day).*

   Following on from no. 8, while many obese people try very hard to
   give the impression that they are happy with their size, healthy,
   never think about it and enjoy a fantastic life, for most of them,
   I believe, this is far from the truth. They would do almost anything
   to be slimmer, but the means of achieving that – possibly hunger,
   deprivation and feeling inferior at the gym or aerobics class – is so
   frightening that it falls outside the realms of 'almost anything'.
   Overweight people are locked, almost frozen, into a status quo
   which keeps them fat. They *do* spend a great deal of time thinking
   about their size and how to get out of the fat trap, but wake up next
   day and once again, nothing changes. The lack of self-confidence
   that makes them eat and want to be invisible is at work here too –
   they simply haven't the confidence to act.

10. *You spend a lot of time compensating for your size. You may be a 'yes'
    person, a people pleaser. You may be the 'life and soul of the party',
    the shoulder for everyone to cry on, the one who always gives way in
    an argument.*

    Low self-esteem is at work here again. Often people who are
    overweight feel the need to be whatever they think will make other
    people like or need them, despite their size.

Even if you ticked most (or all) of the ten key points above, don't feel bad.
Let me repeat – if you are fat or obese, it isn't all your own fault. You may have

contributed to it (by buying the food, eating it, not taking enough exercise), but you have been persuaded, cajoled and bullied by all manner of factors into doing it. You didn't do it on your own.

So let's now take a closer look at all that conspires to get us and keep us overweight.

The Fat-promoters

There are many, many more fat-promoters in your life than you ever would have thought, some disguising themselves as really, really nice people, or pleasures, or perhaps as nice jobs, funky gadgets – oh such a lot.

Food manufacturers and supermarkets

Several years ago, when I was writing *The Diet Bible*, I worked out exactly what it would mean in terms of lost revenue to the food manufacturers of the UK if every adult were to lose a stone in weight. The answer was that the uneaten *seventeen thousand billion* calories would mean a loss of approximately £17 billion in revenue to the food industry.

It's obvious, isn't it, that it is in the interests of every producer, manufacturer and retailer to get us to eat more? That way lies profit. And yet we still fall for it. We still lap up all those buy-one-get-one-free offers.

But our gullibility does not affect only our weight and health, it also lightens our purses and contributes to the world's food shortage problems and environmental issues: every time any one of us eats more than we need to survive and stay a reasonable size and healthy, we are wasting food.

And not only are we wasting the food itself, but the resources needed to make and transport it. Most of the surplus food we eat (snack foods, 'treats', takeaways, ready meals) is highly processed and/or highly energy inefficient. A slice of cake, for example, contains refined wheat, refined fat, is baked, wrapped, stored and transported; a sausage roll contains meat – the production of which is one of the highest users of energy and one of the highest causes of food-related greenhouse gases – and has then been processed using ingredients that include refined flour again, and refined fat again ...

So next time you see a banner or an advertisement which promises that you will 'save money' if you buy this or that, think again. (We will look more closely at how to restore your natural instincts for food and what you really need in Chapter Four.)

It is also no coincidence that much of the food that we think we enjoy eating contains high levels of refined wheat flour, manufactured fats and sugar. Fat, flour and sugar – which account for much of our calorie consumption – are three of the lowest-cost items, providing bulk and calories for little outlay. Indeed, the National Consumer Council has found that over a three-year period, sales of cut-price discount foods and special promotions have increased by 83 per cent, and that these deals are most often for foods high in fats and sugars.

Behind the scenes in the food industry, food scientists are constantly looking for new ways of turning basic produce into something they can sell us – testing different ways to blend fat, flour, sugar and salt to achieve what they term the 'bliss point', whereby food slips down our gullets easily and leaves us wanting more.

Politicians

In the introduction to this book, I referred to a seminar I attended in Whitehall in early 2009 about children and obesity, at which each and every participant claimed to want to solve the prevailing obesity problem.

Sadly, however, a dig into the workings of parliament and government, both in the UK and in the USA, forces me to conclude that, as long as political parties are backed financially and in other ways by the very food manufacturing and distribution companies discussed above, there is no way that the necessary sweeping changes needed in the amount and type of food that is sold to us will take place.

(Incidentally, food companies have also managed to muscle in on what should be unbiased organisations, such as nutrition foundations and medical societies. So action for change at a 'higher level' is always going to be tricky.)

Food caterers

It's hard to believe that just fifty years ago, dining out was a rarity, fast-food outlets were limited to a few pioneer Wimpy burger bars and takeaway meant no choice but fish and chips.

Until the economic recession in 2009, figures were still soaring with people eating out around 100 per cent more than they did twenty years ago, while spending on food and drink consumed outside the home hit £87.5 billion per annum.

While at the more expensive 'luxury' end of the eating-out market (the Michelin-starred restaurants and hotels), the tendency is to serve small portions of foods (often foods low in calories); the lower down the eating-out chain you go, the more likely you are to be buying food that is high in calories, fat and refined carbs and low in plants. From 'pub grub' – the meat pie, the chips, the traditional puddings – through to burger bars, pizza chains, coffee shops and street-corner ethnic takeaways, what you are most likely to be getting is plenty of food for your money (so you feel like it is a bargain), but something that, if you eat it too often and don't take enough exercise to burn it off, will almost certainly put fat on you.

Somehow, while we've been inundated in the past decade or two with information about how to cook healthily at home, how to reduce fat and calories, these basics don't seem to have filtered through to all the people who produce and sell food eaten outside the home. I could count on one hand the number of well-known food outlets serving genuinely healthy meals across their whole menus, as opposed to one or two token 'healthy' offerings among the more popular fat- and calorie-laden choices.

The alcohol industry

Our collective increased intake of alcoholic drinks over the years has, undoubtedly, had an effect on our waistlines. And the drinks industry has as many tricks to encourage us to drink more as the food industry does.

Alcohol is advertised on TV and in the media, it's used for sponsorship and it somehow seems to be glamorous and comforting, confidence-boosting and cool.

Like comfort food, in times of uncertainty and even hardship (such as a global recession), we may spend less on alcohol, but we will consume just as much, especially of the lower-cost brands.

People who use food as a crutch may also be prone to use alcohol in the same way. And because one of the effects of alcohol is to lower self-control, it therefore increases the likelihood that we will eat more than we intended.

Thus, encouraging us to drink alcohol ensures that the battle to remain slim becomes even harder.

Transportation

In the war against fat, the ability to move things quickly and easily around the world is yet another blow.

Put simply, because (thanks to improvements in transport) we have access to more and different foods and can now eat the flavours of the world – we do.

It is proven that if you go to a buffet, laid out with enticing dishes of meats, salads, pastries, cheeses and so on, and are told to eat until you have had enough, you will consume more than if you were to sit down to a meal eaten off a single plate, containing only two or three things, and again told to eat until you have had enough. We eat with our eyes and our senses and we become more greedy when we see a variety of foods in a range of colours.

It is also proven that we like novelty – we want to try as many new foods as we can, while if we are given only familiar foods, we are likely to eat only to satisfy hunger.

Thus, in the early post-war periods in the UK, when the bulk of our diet came from the 'same old' foods such as green and root vegetables, bread, milk and meat and there was little innovation, we weren't tempted to eat more than we needed. We made do with what we had, and thought little about food beyond whether or not there was enough to feed the family and how to make cabbage interesting for the fifth time in any given week.

With this in mind, it will be fascinating to find out if the current interest in 'eating local' and reducing imports will indeed result in a natural tightening of the population's waistbands.

Refrigeration

Going back to the early to mid-1900s, before every household had a fridge and a freezer, we couldn't buy food in large quantities because it would either go stale or off. With the advent of chilling and freezing, however, we found that we could keep a range of foods for much, much longer and thus we could buy more. So we did.

On a commercial level, half of the items on the menus of our cafés and restaurants would not be there without chiller facilities, so menus would be pared down and choice limited. The meat, fish and dairy sections of each and every supermarket would be hard pressed to survive, and ice-cream vans would become a thing of the past.

Packaging

Go back a hundred years or so and most of the food you bought would not have been pre-packed. Flour, sugar, grains, nuts, seeds and pulses, fruit and vegetables would all have been bought loose. Milk would be in bottles (usually from a delivery van) and bread in paper bags.

And so – this is going to sound simplistic, but it's worth pointing out – most of the places where food is sold today, wouldn't be able to sell that food without the packaging industry. It stands to reason that in every supermarket, the vast majority of what is sold is packaged and at least half of what is sold would not be there if it weren't for packaging.

But there is a wider implication. The packaging industry has allowed food, particularly the snack foods and drinks that make a huge mark on our calorie intake – to be sold in all kinds of places that aren't actually designated food outlets. Without packaging, you would not be able to buy cartons of high-calorie soft drinks at service stations; there would be no drink and snack counters at the cinema or theatre; no grabbing a pre-packed sandwich from the coffee counter on the way to work.

As our 'snacking-on-the-hoof' habit has been irrefutably linked with our growth in obesity, it seems reasonable to suggest that the packaging industry has a lot to answer for!

The car

The man who invented the car is normally acknowledged as the German, Karl Benz, who patented the first car back in 1886.

I live 8km (5 miles) from the nearest town with shops. The small road to that town is hilly, very hilly. If I had lived in my house a hundred years ago, I would have had to either walk, cycle or tack up a horse to get to the town – but once there, of course, I would not have found the range of shops there are today, selling all manner of foods (see above). So I would probably have had to grow or rear some of my own food – vegetables, fruit, chickens, ducks; and I would have been happy to go out from spring to autumn and harvest food from the wild – berries, nuts, leaves, stone fruits – or maybe even take a gun and shoot pigeons and rabbits.

All this would have ensured that I kept fit and slim. A 12km (10 mile), three-hour round-trip walk once a week would have burnt up around a thousand calories and been more than equivalent to the amount of exercise that most people get in the UK and USA today during an average week, which is around fifty minutes.

When the car was invented and eventually became more affordable to run, it completely changed our interaction with food and the amount of exercise we take. It has rendered walking as a necessity virtually redundant, especially for those who live in the country, where public transport such as trains, tubes and buses is almost non-existent. People who commute in big towns and cities are better off because at least they get to walk from the train to the office – but even they will usually take the car to the station nearest to their homes.

We used to take a walk, to admire the view, play in the park, on our days off. Now we get in the car, stop the car, take a look at the view, have a vast picnic or cream tea, then get back in the car and head for home. We've replaced activity with inactivity.

The powered lawnmower ...

... and all those other powered tools that mean we burn up far fewer calories doing regular jobs which were once completely reliant on manpower (the vacuum cleaner, washing machine, hedge cutter, to name a few). And at an industrial level, there are the people who were once described as 'manual labourers', but who now simply man powered tools – the JCB, forklift truck etc. Factory jobs of all kinds, with everything automated, are no longer as physical as they were even a few decades ago.

Television

Scot John Logie Baird is often credited with the invention of the television, but other people had a hand in its development. In the latter half of the twentieth century, television proved so fascinating that, almost overnight, people in the Western world stopped pottering around in the evening after work or at the weekends and sat on a sofa, watching a square box for hours instead.

And in more recent years, TV has turned most of us into voyeurs, not doers. When you can see your favourite sport on TV, why go to the match? When you can see the top of Everest or even Snowdon on that wide screen, why get off your bum to go and see it for yourself? Go dancing? Well, yes, but we'd just as soon stay in and watch *Strictly Come Dancing*. Go on a walking holiday to the Lake District? Perhaps – but *Wainwright Walks* on TV has taken away the necessity, somehow.

In its defence, TV can introduce people to hobbies and ideas that they might not otherwise have thought about, and might sometimes encourage people to take up a sport (for example, kids' gymnastics classes and athletics clubs fill to bursting after the Olympics are screened). But it is a fact that before TV was invented, we spent much less of our spare time sitting, just ticking over metabolically, than we do now. And as watching TV advertising also encourages us to eat it can provide two negatives instead of one.

The microchip

Thanks, mainly, to US engineer Jack Kilby, who demonstrated the first microchip circuit technology in 1958, we have another big baddie now, encouraging hours of inactivity. Chatting, gaming, downloading, watching, surfing, listening, emailing – we love our computers. With friends, interests and fun at our fingertips, why ever bother to go out of the home again?

If you happen to have an office job, you'll probably spend all day too, enduring the physical drawbacks of computers and the other trappings of modern working life – using email or phones instead of walking to a meeting, taking lifts and escalators instead of stairs, working through lunch with an order-in meal, rather than strolling or window shopping. While if you work from home at your office job, you don't even get to commute. (I can talk – my office is about six metres from my bedroom door, so some days when I'm really busy, I don't even need to go downstairs, it's just bed to bath to book writing in a few small steps.)

> **FACT**
> In a 2009 UK Department of Health survey of over a quarter of a million families, it was found that around half of all children spend several hours every day in front of the TV and computer, while only one fifth do any form of physical activity.

In conclusion, yes, modern life – our life – is configured to make our figures fatter. And it is a determined individual who goes against the grain, who eats until he or she has had just enough, and who keeps properly active. I can do no better than to quote a Foresight report on the subject of obesity and health:

> The obesity epidemic cannot be prevented by individual action alone and demands a societal approach. Tackling obesity requires far greater change than anything tried so far, and at multiple levels: personal, family, community and national.
>
> Preventing obesity is a societal challenge, similar to climate change. It requires partnership between government, science, business and civil society.

I did say it wasn't your fault you're fat. And now you can see why. But let's take the next step now and see just what can be done about it.

3
The Truth About Your Ideal Body

Our obsession with scales, weighing, Body Mass Index (BMI), growth charts for children and so on is a fairly modern phenomenon. In fact, bathroom scales weren't even invented until the 1940s, and before then, people didn't really know what they weighed unless they put a penny in a public weighing machine. And they got by. If they felt OK, looked OK, didn't look too different from most other people and could fit into their clothes, then all was fine.

So is there actually an 'ideal' weight, below or above which we should begin to panic?

The answer is, no. Not really. What there is, is an 'ideal weight range' for our height (BMI), supplied to us by statisticians who have analysed what populations weigh and produced charts based on averages. If we believe what they tell us, in any event, even the parameters of an ideal weight give us around 12 kilograms' (a couple of stone) leeway in which to enjoy life.

However, our bodies, naturally, change in weight and shape as we age. From birth to death, there are several different weights which may be 'ideal' at any given time, depending upon how old we are and, possibly, other factors.

And, just to confuse things further, there are several experts who disagree with the concept of an ideal weight range, in any case, and who have statistics which they believe prove that good health is not always linked with 'ideal' weight.

So where does that leave you and I? Let's see.

Negotiating the Weight Maze

Body Mass Index

We'll start with another look at those much-discussed and often derided Body Mass Index charts. These were compiled originally for life insurance companies who had discovered a link between weight and life span. Their statistics showed that people who were obese were likely to die younger than people who weren't, and thus obese people had to pay more for their life cover.

The link between health and a 'good weight' is probably correct. There is certainly a huge amount of scientific and statistical evidence showing a connection between all the major diseases of our modern world (heart disease, diabetes and cancer for example) and obesity. But in the case of simple overweight – that is a BMI higher than 'normal', but not high enough to be classified as obese – the evidence is less clear and this brings on the debate about what your own 'good' weight should be.

BODY MASS INDEX (BMI)
BMI = Your weight in kilograms divided by your height in metres squared
How the results are classified:

Under 18.5	underweight
18.5–under 25	normal weight range
25–under 30	overweight
30–under 35	obese class 1
35–under 40	obese class 2
40 and over	obese class 3 (morbidly obese)

Note: for under-18s, there is a different formula, depending on the person's age/height/weight.

∗ *What the BMI proponents say*
- It is the best and most reliable tool we have for measuring and comparing adult weight; it is also cost-free and easily worked out by everyone.
- While it can be inaccurate, for 99 per cent of the population it is not.
- An individual's weight is important because overweight, obesity and underweight are all linked with a variety of health problems and even life-threatening issues.

∗ *What the BMI detractors say*
- It is not an accurate gauge of a person's body fat percentage, a high level of which is more significant than being overweight.
- One often-quoted example is of the professional body-builder or field athlete. Even though he/she may have a body fat percentage much

lower than the average, on the scales he or she will probably register a BMI in the overweight category. The reason for this is a high lean tissue percentage (muscle) which weighs more than fat or bone.

- BMI also takes no account of body-fat distribution – one person with a BMI of, say, 26, may have much surplus fat around the waist, while another may carry more of it on the hips and thighs. Body-fat distribution may be as significant, or more so, than either total weight or total body fat. Not only is a large waist a health risk factor, so is the amount of internal body fat you carry (around the organs and inside your stomach – visceral fat, as opposed to subcutaneous fat, under the skin).

✻ *What I say*
All the 'pros' and 'cons' above are true.

BMI is, for most of us, a great way of getting a rough idea of whether or not we have a weight issue. At either end of the BMI – very low or very high – you can be relatively sure that you do have a problem. For example, if your BMI is 40, you are seriously obese, and fat distribution is almost immaterial. As for athletes and people who, for whatever reason, have a very high lean-tissue percentage, they will almost always know this for themselves – they are likely to be fit, with good body appearance and thus the argument about BMI inaccuracy in this instance is really academic.

It is, however, in the middle range that the picture becomes less clear. The ideal BMI of between 18.5 and 25 is all well and good. But in the range from 23 up to 27 or 28, your body-fat distribution may indeed be more important than your actual weight and BMI. Depending upon what that is, you could be a very healthy person with a BMI of 28, or an at-risk person with a BMI at 23–25, the top end of the 'normal' range. In other words, the classification of BMI between 25 and 30 as 'overweight' and unhealthy is risky. This was backed up by a 2008 study published in the *International Journal of Epidemiology* which monitored 76,000 people for over a decade. It found that a BMI of 25–27.4 had no statistically significant link with increased risk of death.

Other ways of deciding ideal weight

✻ *Waist circumference*
Let me give you a good example of someone who, although falling within the normal/ideal BMI, may be at risk of health problems because of her body-fat distribution: me.

I have a BMI of 24, which is within the healthy range. I keep my weight around 6kg (1 stone) higher than it used to be when I was younger because of a family history of osteoporosis (more of which later; see p. 45). However, I am an apple shape, meaning that my hips are fairly slim, but my body fat wants to congregate, unfairly and visibly, around my middle. And so my waist measurement hovers dangerously near the upper limit for safety in a woman, which is why I have to be careful about taking regular exercise – the only way I have found to keep my waistline down. If I had less fat around my middle and more on my hips (a pear shape), I could have a BMI higher than 24 – nearer to 27 or 28 – and I would probably be less at risk of health problems due to my weight/shape/body fat than I am now.

'Central fat distribution', as the apple phenomenon is called, is definitely linked with an increased risk of a variety of problems. In 2008, Harvard Medical School reported on the study of 44,000 nurses that showed even normal-weight women are at increased risk of death from heart disease and cancer if they are larger than average around the midriff. And this is just one of many similar studies.

So, when considering whether or not you should lose weight, it is quite important to take your shape – your measurement around your middle – into account, as well as your actual weight. If you find that your waist is over 81cm (32in) for women or 95cm (37.5in) for men, it is probably time to take steps to reduce it (see box below, for more details).

WAIST CIRCUMFERENCE CHART

	You are at risk	You are at high risk
If your waist is over (women):	81cm (32in)	88cm (35in)
(men):	94cm (37.5in)	102cm (41in)

---

* Mirror test

Another way to gauge a good weight for you is to look at yourself, naked, in a full-length mirror:

- If you see folds of fat and skin anywhere, particularly around the middle, you are likely to be overweight.
- If you see your belly sticking out further than your chest when you turn sideways, you are, again, likely to be overweight, or at least in need of changes to diet and exercise regimes.

- If you have a large middle (see chart, above), but slim, undefined arms and legs, then you are also likely to be overweight and in need of the right forms of exercise. With such a shape, it could well be that your BMI is perfect (22–24) because your limbs weigh less than average and this is offsetting the extra weight around your middle.
- If you see none of the above, but a fairly firm-looking body, possibly with large hips and sturdy thighs, but with little or no flab around the midriff and some waist definition, then even though you may come in with a BMI at the top end of ideal or in the overweight category, it is probable that your weight is causing you no health problems at all.

✱ Gadgets

There are various gadgets you can buy which claim to give you an accurate reading of your body fat, and you can also go to gyms/clinics for weight and/or body fat assessment, which will cost you more. None of this is really necessary. A commonsense assessment of your own BMI, coupled with the waist circumference test and the mirror test (above) should tell you what you need to know. However, I do look at the available gadgets and tests for sale in more detail, in Chapter Seven.

Weight and Health –
How Clear Is the Picture?

There are some actual advantages to having a reasonable amount of body fat, especially for women, as I explained in Chapter One. It helps to insulate our bodies and protect our bones; it produces the hormone leptin, which boosts the immune system and can help to enhance our mood; it is vital for fertility and reproduction, and vital during and after the menopause to help boost oestrogen activity and to protect against osteoporosis.

I would describe a 'reasonable amount' of body fat as at least the amount present in someone in the upper to normal range of BMI – about 24/5, and for pear-shaped people (with a defined waistline), even as high as 26/7, especially pre-, during and post-menopause.

Recent findings from a study run by scientists at Oxford University into a million British women back this up. They found that the ideal BMI for health in females is 24. While a 2007 report published in the *American Journal of Public*

Health found that the ideal BMI for men is 26 – at that level males have the highest life expectancy of all. So the advantages of a covering of body fat may not be restricted to women.

The 'healthy weight' debate is muddied by the fact that you can't isolate a person's weight and link it conclusively with their good or ill health because there are other factors that need to be taken into consideration:

- Does an obese person have heart disease because he is obese, for example, or because he eats a poor diet high in trans fats and sugar and low in fruit and vegetables (i.e. heart-protective vitamins, minerals and compounds)?
- Is a slim, vegan person healthy and likely to live a long life because she is slim, or because she eats more than the 'allotted' five portions of fruit and vegetables a day and no high-fat dairy, or cancer-inducing chargrilled meat?
- Does the very thin person have a heart condition because of her borderline anorexia and nutrient deficiencies, or because she smokes thirty cigarettes a day to keep herself thin?

Research has found that vegetarians do tend to be slimmer and live longer than meat-eaters. But when you examine the lifestyles of vegetarians and vegans, you find that as well as eating a non-meat diet, they also tend to exercise more than non-vegetarians and are less likely to smoke, take drugs or drink alcohol – all or some of which may be the real reason they live longer, rather than the fact that they weigh less.

Headline stories – what should you believe?

I'm going to digress now slightly, to look at what the newspapers and magazines have to say on weight/health. This will help you to find your way through the whole issue and to exercise a healthy amount of scepticism when reading the latest weight/health/fitness news and apply it to your growing body intelligence.

The stories that are particularly suspect are those that are based on low-number population studies. This is when a group of researchers look at segments of the population (sometimes of more than one country, other times just a few people in a particular town, occupation or so on) over time – perhaps a few weeks, perhaps a year or several years – and draw conclusions from what they discover.

These studies may rely on self-reporting from the participants. For example, if the study is about whether people who regularly eat ice cream suffer from more indigestion than people who don't, the participants need to remember to record *every time* they eat ice cream and they need to be truthful. They also need to do the same for their bouts of indigestion. This gives plenty of room for error in the individual studies and in the results of the report. It is also hard to prove that it was the ice cream that caused the indigestion – it could have been the cheese eaten before the ice cream, for example.

However, the report will still be published and the papers will still sensationalise its 'findings'. The result being a headline that reads: 'Ice cream killer: those who eat ice cream are fifty times more likely to suffer from chronic digestive problems than those who don't!'

An overview – in which a group of researchers analyse all the studies that have been conducted on a particular subject, put them all through the computer and come up with an overview of the results – is another form of research. It can have a few advantages over the smaller, localised report, in that while it can't take out the errors that may have been in the original reports, it does tend to 'smooth out' the findings and can take account of the size of the original reports. (For example, were ten people or a million people involved in the study? If there were a million, the results carry considerably more weight than if there were ten.) Thus findings from overviews may be more useful than those from small or random studies.

Overviews are also conducted on scientific trial reports. Scientific trials are those (unlike population studies) that have involved proper, double-blind experiments under laboratory conditions. For example (and this is a fictional one!): if fifty human volunteers are each given 25g (1oz) butter to eat and their blood fat levels shoot up by an average of 100 per cent within 30 minutes, the researchers may draw the conclusion that eating butter can increase short-term blood fat levels by 100 per cent. For a double-blind trial, there should also be a 'control group' – in this case, fifty volunteers who are given 25g of something other than butter (the dummy), to compare the butter results against without knowing whether they were eating butter or the dummy.

So you can rely on scientific trial reports ... maybe. Sometimes. Like population studies, they may be conducted on just a few people, and if the results are marginal (say, blood fat levels only increased after butter ingestion by 5 per cent, and the trial only involved twenty people, not fifty), the results would be less conclusive. Results can also vary according to the participants involved. For example, the experiment might produce a different result using people who are prone to high blood cholesterol as opposed to people whose blood cholesterol is normal. Experiments may also be conducted on animals, not humans, and while lab rats and mice are similar to humans in many ways, and initial research carried out on them may indeed later be replicated on humans, that isn't always the case. But the media scaremongers will bury the fact that the trial is small, the results marginal or the whole thing done on animals, two thirds of the way into the story and you just might miss it.

Another thing to look out for is whether or not the research was sponsored by an interested party – a report on anti-wrinkle cream or cellulite treatment sponsored by a cosmetic company, for example; or a report claiming to show that salt is not linked to high blood pressure, sponsored by a salt manufacturer. That is not to say the results are false, but they could be analysed in such a way that they say what the sponsors want them to say.

For example, you might read a headline that claims, 'Likelihood of kidney stones increases by 200 per cent if you are overweight'. But if you look at the actual study, you might find that the volunteers are all at least 32kg (5 stone) overweight, that in the healthy control group there is only one case of kidney stones in 1000, but that in the test group that rises to two in 1000. Thus, even for severely overweight people, the chances of them contracting kidney stones would be a mere one in 500. The headline could almost just as well be, 'Overweight has little effect on incidence of kidney stones'!

So, when deciding on the significance or otherwise of any new report, remember the following:

- Look at the number and type of people involved.
- Look at the actual figures/results of the experiment or trial.
- Ignore the headlines.

As I said, a healthy amount of scepticism is a vital ingredient of body intelligence. Oh, and by the way – if I quote medical, research or scientific studies in this book, I tend to use the largest studies and only those whose results have been verified and published in reputable scientific journals!

When Weight DOES Matter

Although the whole business of weight and how much being 'normal weight' actually matters is fudged with doubt and disagreement, there are some irrefutable facts and possibly inconvenient truths and probabilities that I can record.

Weight and health/life span/wellbeing

Obesity – a BMI of over 30 – is what the World Health Organisation describes as a 'chronic disease and a growing threat' in itself. The National Audit Office says obesity causes at least 30,000 deaths a year in the UK. Hospital admissions for weight-related problems increase by around 30 per cent year on year and in 2008, no fewer than 1.2 million drug prescriptions to control the epidemic were written. Obesity is very strongly linked with a range of individual health problems and diseases:

- **Cancer** Each year approximately 13,000 people in the UK develop cancer because they are overweight/obese, according to Cancer Research UK. And in 2009, the World Cancer Research Fund found that over a third of cancers were related to poor diet and lack of exercise. Overweight is most strongly linked with cancers of the uterus, breast, kidney, bowl and oesophagus. The reason for this link is that excess body fat is metabolically active – it produces a surplus of cancer-causing hormones.
- **Cardiovascular (CV) disease** This is strongly linked with obesity, with data produced over several decades supporting the connection between the two. In particular, central fat distribution (apple shape, see p. 44) increases the risk by more than 40 per cent. High blood pressure – a risk factor for CV disease – is three times more prevalent in overweight people than non-overweight. Obesity is also strongly associated with a poor blood-fats profile – for example, reduced levels of 'good' HDL cholesterol and raised levels of 'bad' LDL cholesterol.
- **Type 2 diabetes** Around 70 per cent of cases are in overweight and obese people and, once more, this is linked to the 'apple-shape' body more than to the 'pear shape'. Reduction in weight and an increase in activity can cure type 2 diabetes in a significant proportion of sufferers.
- **Arthritis** Symptoms of osteoarthritis, back and joint pain are all made worse by overweight, as extra strain is placed on the joints.
- **Asthma and breathing problems, including sleep apnoea** These are made worse by obesity as internal body fat obstructs the airways.
- **Pregnancy complications** Obesity in pregnancy increases the risk of pregnancy complications, a Caesarean delivery and stillbirth.
- **Loss of mobility** Obese people are less likely than average to take regular exercise – indeed often they are unable to exercise due to

linked problems such as arthritis, breathing difficulties or heart disease. Lack of exercise itself is linked with most of the health problems listed above.

- **Brain power** Reducing food intake by around 30 per cent has been shown to dramatically improve memory in females. While this does not actually prove that obesity lowers brain power, there is plenty of evidence to show that a healthy diet and body weight can increase concentration and various aspects of brain function and may protect against Alzheimer's disease.

So it is hardly surprising that large population studies have shown a direct correlation between obesity and early death. For instance, the huge USA Nurses Health Study (an ongoing USA study of over 200,000 nurses, begun in 1976) showed that in female nurses, the relative risk of overall mortality increased virtually exactly in line with increased weight. And another study of 1 million US adults of all ages showed an increased risk in death from all causes in people ranging from moderately to severely overweight. Lastly, a recent overview of all the studies carried out by Oxford University in 2009 found that a BMI of between 30 and 35 reduced survival by two to four years, while a BMI over 40 reduced it by eight to ten years.

I believe the point to reiterate here is that, in most cases, disease and early death are linked with BMI over 30, and that while at BMIs of around 27–30 there may be an increased risk of health problems, this is much more likely if you have central fat distribution.

So, if you're plump but not obese – watch the belly!

Work

Sometimes your weight and shape will hold you back from the life you want. A 2009 study found that women, in particular, suffer from fat discrimination in the workplace, being less likely to 'get the job' after an interview and less likely to get promotion. Government figures show that over 2000 people are claiming benefits because their obesity is preventing them from finding work; but this is just the tip of the iceberg, as there are millions of lost working days due to size-related illness.

Economy and ecology

As we have seen, obesity costs the UK economy a great deal. The National Audit Office estimates that obesity costs the economy as a whole £2 billion, and the

NHS in particular, at least £500 million a year to treat. If each and every one of us was to maintain a reasonable weight, the burden on the NHS would be considerably lower.

As I pointed out in my book *The Green Food Bible*, back in 2007, one way of helping the environment and the beckoning threat of worldwide food shortages due to increasing populations and global warming is to consume fewer calories, i.e. less food. That would mean more food to go around, less energy expended in food production, transport costs, packaging and so on. We would also all save money – not only on food bills, but also, in some cases, on liposuction and other cosmetic procedures that deal with the effects of overeating.

Being too fat is not environmentally friendly. So if you are a 'green', add watching your waistline to your list of energy-saving measures.

Your personal life

Marital, sexual and social life can all be negatively affected or even destroyed by weight issues. Obese people are less likely to find partners or to lead an active sexual life and more prone than others to spending long periods at home, rather than interacting with other people. In other words, obese people are more likely than not to be unfulfilled in several areas of their lives.

And When It Doesn't

You may not like your shape, but unless your body is putting you at risk in terms of health, the bits you dislike are aesthetically, not clinically, important. For example, you may think your thighs are too fat, your knees too chubby or bony, your feet too big, your neck too short, your bust too small or a hundred other things I've heard from friends and acquaintances. But none of these things really matters; indeed, most of them are probably things that no one but you would ever even notice.

When we looked at the cult of skinny in Chapter One, I said that there is no such thing as a perfect body. Even men and women who are idolised by others for their 'perfection' will, if you get to know them, reveal insecurities about their looks and things they would change if they could.

I once spent a few hours with a group of naturists (nudists) at their weekly meeting at a health club. I went along out of curiosity about how it would feel, how they would be, and I was very glad I did. At the time, I had quite a 'good' body – slim-ish, not flabby; I remember the only thing I worried about was my skin being too white, rather than tanned.

What I remember most about the experience are the different shapes and sizes, mostly variations of 'normal' – some fatter, some thinner, but all individual, and not one person with what you might describe as the body beautiful. Yet nobody there was worried about the way they looked. They were all naturists for their own different reasons, but I was struck by how relaxed, cheerful and confident they were. Not exhibitionist, yet not minding their vulnerability, with nothing to hide behind except their own skin.

I am not sure what this proves except that perhaps what matters most about you and your body is improving your own relationship with what you have, so that you too could pop along to the naturist beach or club and not worry one jot what you look like.

I also keep in mind the people I have known who, for one reason or another, lost their health or their strength: my friends Peter and Buck, who both developed cancer at a young age and faded away from life; my mother, who physically almost vanished, as she aged into her eighties and nineties; my friend Coral, who has an amazing brain and the will to do almost anything in life – but a pain-ridden body that just won't do the things she wants it to do; my sister, who has multiple sclerosis and battles to overcome her difficulties and live a normal life; my sister-in law, fighting breast cancer as I write. Even myself – diagnosed out of the blue with malignant melanoma six years ago, followed by a year of operations and hospital visits, then finally, and thankfully, the all-clear, five years on.

All of us who lose our health and strength regret the same things: not having been thankful enough for a fit body when we had one; having taken wellness, strength, fitness and health for granted; and having moaned and quibbled about our imperfections.

It is important to embrace your shape and enjoy its benefits, while understanding what you can – or should – change or adapt, and how to do so in a manner designed for long-term success and health. The remainder of this chapter discusses how you can go about doing that.

Ideals and Realities ...

... or achievables and non-achievables.

We all cheat a bit, some of the time – pulling the tummy in, wearing make-up, dying our hair, wearing black. Torture underwear, however (you know, those garments that strap you in from above the knee to below the bust, take an age to put on and are meant to make you feel better about yourself but, actually, highlight the fact that you are desperate) is, to me, one cheat too far. It is akin to cosmetic surgery – simply, not being kind to yourself.

What you really need to achieve is a body you can feel comfortable and healthy in, and whether you get that just by changing it until you are comfortable, or by adjusting the way you feel about it, if the changes aren't actually necessary for your health and wellbeing, that's fine. The points below (some of which have been covered earlier in the chapter in more detail) should help you to decide what you can change, how you might change and whether change is even necessary or desirable. Acknowledging them is one of the keys to body IQ, and they may be the most important body facts you'll read:

Four things you need to know about your body ... and why they are important

* *The basic shape you are as a young adult is the basic shape you will be for most of your life.*
You can alter the 'cladding' on your body (e.g. you can get a bust enlargement, liposuction to get a smaller waist or lose or gain fat, or, to some extent, muscle). But if you have wide hips and a narrow waist and back, you will always be pear-shaped. Your basic shape is based on bone structure and hardly alters until you are much older when shape changes are noticeable due to reduced bone mass and fluid depletion.
Conclusion: Be aware of your shape (as I said earlier it is important if you are apple-shaped to be wary of developing fat around your middle), but accept what's achievable and what isn't, and be realistic about which parts of your body you can change through diet and exercise.

* *Fitness is more important than weight.*
While a top-class, long-distance runner is almost certain to have a low BMI, they will have excellent cardiovascular fitness. A top model, by contrast, also with a low BMI, will be much less likely to be fit. Most female models take little exercise, keep their weight low by smoking and minimal food intake and have poor muscle definition (easy to spot as arms and legs are thin and shapeless).
Conclusion: Large numbers of women who have spent years keeping their weight low by means of diet alone may be at risk of ill health. It is important to increase activity and general fitness to maintain a healthy weight rather than focus on slimness.

* *Dieting can be one of the worst things you can do for your body, your health and your shape.*
Millions of women across the world have done their bodies absolutely no favours by spending much of their lives dieting. Repeated low-calorie diets,

repeated weight loss and weight gain (especially coupled with a lack of exercise) ensure that, over the years, it becomes harder and harder to lose weight and more likely that you will regain it once lost. This is mainly because repeated diets shed lean tissue, which tends not to be replaced (partly because you don't eat much protein and partly because you don't do exercise to build and maintain muscle); thus, with each new diet, the metabolic rate tends to decline. Repeated diets are also linked with increased risk of heart disease, poor blood-fat profile, weakening of the immune system and nutritional deficiencies, as well as with a loss of self-esteem and other negative emotions.

Conclusion: There are no miracle quick fixes as far as weight control goes. Like the tortoise and the hare, being sensible and taking it slowly works best.

✱ *It is easier to achieve a better body using methods you enjoy.*
We can all do things we don't want to do for short periods of time – whether it is studying, washing up or avoiding some of the foods we like best. But it is more pleasant and easier to achieve what we want using methods that don't depress or annoy us. Yet 90 per cent of people who decide they want to lose weight or get fit, do so using methods they don't really like, or even actively dislike. And down that route lies ultimate failure.

Conclusion: Motivation and goals are important and can carry your plans and you a long way and, in the short term, can help to overcome the negative aspects of your task. For example, if you want to slim down for a special occasion, you may be able to ignore hunger and boredom and live on juice and cabbage soup for a week. But for long-term success you need actively to enjoy what you're doing.

In conclusion, I cannot stress strongly enough that you will never be happy with your body unless you accept its unalterable idiosyncrasies, as well as a limit on how much you can accomplish with the alterable imperfections.

It is more important to achieve something, and then enjoy that achievement in the long term, than to feel continually frustrated, trying to get somewhere that's too hard to reach, or abusing your body in the quest.

However, it is also important to be honest – to face up to the truth if, indeed, you are life-threateningly overweight, rather than to insist you simply have heavy bones or sluggish glands.

The next section of the book – Body IQ – looks at what IS honest and true. We'll be looking at all the ways people try to tame their bodies, and what really works. We will begin with the most-often cited diet myths – the tales that have become accepted as reality over the years – and examine the truth behind them.

Part Two:
Body IQ

4
Myths and Truths
A Closer Look at Food and Weight Control

We all know the person who analyses each meal, each mouthful, for its calorie or fat content, who refuses all carbs, dairy, meat and so on because they are 'bad for you', or they say they have an allergy or intolerance. We know the person who obsesses about tiny bits of fat on their plate. We may even be that person.

But can we blame them? We are all constantly bombarded with information coming at us from all sides. There are newspapers which might say one thing about diet on page 5 and the exact opposite in a feature on page 15. There are internet sites which appear to be sensible and helpful, but which peddle rubbish 'facts' in order to sell us something. There are doctors, nutritionists, practitioners, laymen and goodness knows who else trying to make a living out of our gullibility. And there are journalists and media people who take shortcuts when writing articles and add 'facts' to their features without checking them.

In this chapter, I aim to set the record straight about the 'wisdom' that has come to be carved in stone about dieting, weight control and healthy eating, as well as behaviours connected with all three. I've selected my 'top' bugbears that I hear repeated time and again – most of which are likely to cause more harm than good in your quest for a better body. Although other myths are dispelled throughout the book, the ones I've chosen to focus on in this chapter point up the manner in which we constantly fool ourselves around weight and food topics.

Food: Myths and Truths

False: eating carbs and proteins at the same meal will make you fat

Even a basic school-level knowledge of the digestive system and how our bodies process the food we eat shows that this premise (as in diets such as the Hay system or 'food combining', a method which has sold millions of books) has no scientific basis whatsoever. The originator, William Hay, believed that eating 'foods that fight' caused a build-up of acid toxins in the body followed by disease. However, intended as a disease prevention rather then a weight loss diet, obesity wasn't one of the diseases he had in mind.

* *The truth*
  - Our bodies are designed to digest protein and carbs at the same meal. For thousands of years, even when we ate a stone-age diet of berries, nuts and seeds, we have eaten a diet that contains both.
  - Many carbohydrate foods are a mixture of both protein and carbohydrate (and, often, fat), so avoiding eating both at the same time is actually harder than it might seem. For example, potatoes are about 11 per cent protein, rice is about 8 per cent protein, bread is about 14 per cent protein and lentils are about 30 per cent protein.
  - Food reaches the stomach within seconds of being chewed and swallowed. There, with the help of the gastric juices, it is mostly turned into 'chyme' – a semi-liquid which can then be 'sorted' depending on content. The carbohydrate content of the stomach is processed most quickly – after around two hours it moves down the digestive tract where it mixes with digestive juices and the bulk of absorption of nutrients takes place. Protein is processed the next fastest and fat is slowest of all.
  - However, just because these three major nutrients are processed at different rates, doesn't mean the body finds this a difficult task. And it certainly doesn't make us fat.

False: eating carbs in the evening will make you fat

This may well sound logical – kill the pasta, potatoes and bread after 5 p.m., otherwise they'll sit around in your digestive system while you're asleep and turn to fat. Or something like that.

With no carbs, most people will be drastically cutting the calorie content of their main meal of the day – the evening meal – and thus will lose weight. But …

* *The truth*
This is just another faddy way to restrict calories, with no scientific basis, and, as such, it is not a good long-term strategy. Evenings are the ideal time to relax and enjoy food, and imposing a ban on a major part of most meals is, at best, foolish.

It is also not a good idea because carbs eaten in the evening (if they are the right carbs, see p. 83) can help you sleep well. Good-quality carbs in the evening are a good idea, not a bad one.

False: meat is fattening because it takes so long to digest

I have read various rumours that red meat can 'stay in your body' for years, and because of this, it will make you fat.

✻ *The truth*
Meat *does* take longer to digest than various other foods, such as refined carbohydrates. It is a protein food containing varying levels of fat – and both of these take longer to digest than starches (see p.58). This, if you are trying to lose or maintain weight, is a *good* thing. It means you will be sated for longer than you would with many types of non-meat meal, your blood sugar levels will remain stable and you won't be rushing to the biscuit tin soon after a meal. (This is why so many vegetarians crave sweet foods – they need to be extra careful to replace meat with enough good-quality protein at every meal.)

That said, if you are a long-term vegetarian and then take up meat-eating again, it may take longer for your body to digest meat to begin with. According to Professor David Levitsky of Cornell University, USA, the levels of enzymes that digest meat can fall over time without meat in the diet, but these levels will recover within a few days.

Also, length of digestion time has little bearing on whether a food ends up as fat on your body for people in normal health. A 200-calorie steak can't suddenly become a 300-calorie steak in your body, even if it takes a while to digest. The only way meat may make you fat is if you eat too much of it, particularly fatty cuts, or have it with things like pastry or slathered in cream. However, there is reliable evidence to suggest that a diet high in lean protein (such as lean cuts of meat) can actually help to keep you slim (for more on this, see Chapter Five).

False: eating lots of fruit is the best way to slim

I know a lot of people – women, in particular – who have a 'sweet tooth' and who swap their high-cal sugary snacks, such as biscuits, cakes and chocolate, for a high-fruit diet to lose weight. This may indeed result in a good overall calorie reduction and weight loss – most fruits are low-calorie, high in water and also contain nutrients, such as vitamin C, and some dietary fibre. However – the best way to slim? I think not.

✱ *The truth*

Most fruits are high in a type of sugar called fructose (fruit sugar). Regular high-fructose intake has recently been linked with abdominal fat and an increased likelihood of diabetes, obesity and heart disease. Indeed, it is possible that fructose is worse than sucrose or glucose in this respect.

A University of California study in 2009 found that fructose-sweetened drinks adversely affect both sensitivity to the hormone insulin and the way in which the body handles fats, creating medical conditions that increase susceptibility to heart attack and stroke. In the ten-week study, overweight and obese people consumed glucose- or fructose-sweetened beverages that provided 25 per cent of their daily calories. Both groups put on about the same amount of weight, but only those drinking fructose-sweetened beverages exhibited an increase in intra-abdominal fat, as well as 200 per cent higher blood-fat (triglyceride) levels. People who were already insulin resistant (often termed the pre-diabetic state and associated with obesity and heart disease) had the worst blood-fat results of all.

True, fructose as an added ingredient is not the same as fructose in whole fruit, but the results are interesting. Also, many fruits have a high glycaemic index (GI) profile – a measure of how rapidly carbohydrates are absorbed into the bloodstream – whereby a high GI means that food is rapidly absorbed and may leave you feeling hungry again quickly. A high-GI diet is also linked with obesity, diabetes and abdominal fat. (See p. 85 for more information on the glycaemic index.)

The best way to eat fruit is as part of a meal containing protein and fat to slow down absorption and, in effect, turn the fruit into a low-GI food. Or, interestingly, there is research to show that eating a low GI fruit just before a meal can help, too. The journal *Appetite* published a study in which people who ate an apple fifteen minutes before a meal ate 15 per cent fewer calories. Of course, that would only be of benefit if the 15 per cent reduction was greater than the number of calories in the apple (around sixty).

While fruit is a legitimate part of a healthy diet, the fact is that eating a lot of fruit is not the best way to lose weight. You could do it very well on a diet of lean protein and vegetables which, recent research shows, could have a much better effect on your blood fats and stomach circumference (more about which in Chapter Five).

If you are going to eat a lot of fruit (more than two portions a day), the best to choose are whole fruits, and preferably those with a low GI, such as apples, oranges, pears and cherries. These will have a less damaging effect on your blood-sugar levels and help to prevent hunger from returning quickly.

Note: fruit juice – recommended by so many dieticians as a good addition to any slimmer's daily menu – is, in my opinion, best avoided by slimmers and, indeed, by most people. Without the dietary fibre and the structure of the whole fruit, it is a high-GI, fructose-rich, tooth-rotting nightmare.

False: dairy should be avoided if you want to lose weight

One of the things I hear most frequently from people is that 'dairy' is a real baddie. The most often cited reasons are: 'It is very high in fat', 'It is very high in calories' and 'I am allergic to it'.

✱ The truth

Yes, a lot of dairy produce is high in both fat and calories, and can also be a major source of saturated fat. Too much cream, butter, full-fat cheese (such as Cheddar, cream cheese and Stilton) will not only contribute far too many calories to your diet, but the fat (and in some cases, salt) content could also contribute to health problems, including heart disease.

But as long as you choose your dairy with care (the lower-fat cheeses, milks and yogurts can all be good choices), you should go ahead and enjoy it.

- Believe it or not, quite a lot of scientific research has found a link between regular dairy intake and weight *loss*, not gain! As I explained in Chapter Three, scientific research can be a bit of a minefield because trials involving just ten people can sometimes get as much media coverage as those involving 100,000 people. And, in the case of the dairy/obesity link, trials have varied in size and duration enormously, and results have been mixed. But there seems to me to be enough evidence linking the mineral calcium (of which dairy is a major source) with decreased fat absorption from the diet and increased fat excretion (via the faeces) from the body, to make it worth including low-fat dairy in your diet. One Swiss trial found that adding calcium to chocolate when it is being made reduced the actual calories absorbed in the chocolate by 10 per cent because of this effect.
- Most low-fat cheese is high in protein and low in starches. A high-protein diet has benefits, in that it improves satiety as part of a reduced-calorie diet and improves the regulation of blood-sugar levels and, as several studies have shown, it may help to speed the metabolic rate.

- Yogurt (the natural 'bio' kind) contains probiotic bacteria which have recently also been linked (in trials on pregnant women) with a decrease in 'central obesity' – i.e. stomach fat.

Lastly, a word about the fast-growing number of people who are, apparently, allergic to dairy produce. Yes, some people are allergic to dairy – usually the lactose in milk. But, in my experience, a lot of women who have never been properly tested for, or diagnosed with, a lactose, dairy or milk allergy, avoid dairy nevertheless, citing an allergy. Anyone who thinks they may be allergic or intolerant should go to their GP and ask for a test, and avoid the many thousands of so-called allergy-testing clinics which advertise on the internet and elsewhere. (For more on bogus clinics and practitioners, see Chapter Eight).

False: wheat should be avoided if you want to lose weight

Wheat has had a very bad press for many years in the USA and UK. Bread, pastry, pasta, cake, breakfast cereals are often the first thing to go from the diet of a 'clued-up' female who wants to lose weight. It is not a joke that many carb-phobic Californians will ask for a sandwich – without the bread! The idea is that many of us are wheat-intolerant, and that it is hard to digest, causes bloating and weight problems.

✴ *The truth*
A diet high in simple carbs – of which refined 'white' wheat is one – can cause the body to retain more fluid than a low-carb one, because, in simple terms, the carbs act a bit like 'blotting paper', retaining extra fluid while they go through the digestive system. A test of this is to have a high-carb day, followed by a low-carb day; you will find yourself going to the loo much more on your low-carb day, as the retained fluid is released.

However, fluid is not fat. Wheat, per se, is not that high in calories, and wholegrain wheat is a perfectly good addition to the diet of most people, whether they are slimming or not. That said, bread – both wholemeal and white – is a fairly high-GI food and, if eaten in quantity or without the GI-reducing effects of an accompanying protein/fat food, can affect blood sugars (see p. 69) which may have an indirect effect on weight control. Dark rye and oat breads are better choices as they have a lower GI.

I believe that people who give up wheat, then rave about how much weight they've lost, have benefited not from giving up the wheat, but from eating fewer calories. While bread is not, in itself, a high-calorie food, it is easy to cut yourself a much heavier piece than you would credit. Wheat flour also presents itself in many high-sugar and/or high-fat foods which add little nutritional value to the average diet, but plenty of calories.

A combination of these reasons, or some of them is, I am sure, why people who give up wheat, or cut down drastically, may lose weight and feel better.

So could you be allergic to wheat? About one in 1500 of the UK population is coeliac, meaning they are allergic to the gluten in wheat (and some other grains), causing inflammation of the intestines and serious symptoms, such as malnutrition and anaemia. Allergy to other parts of the wheat grain is very rare. 'Wheat intolerance' isn't a recognised medical condition (one common professional view is that this so-called intolerance is actually a psychological aversion), so official figures of this condition aren't to be found.

False: some foods have negative calories

Over several years, I have had many requests from slimmers for the truth about so-called negative-calorie foods. The premise is that some foods make the digestive system work so hard that more calories are burned up by digestion than the foods actually contain. Therefore, as you eat you lose weight, and the more negative calorie foods you eat, the more weight you lose.

✱ *The truth*
The only thing which may cause a negative energy input/output is ice-cold water! That's because if you drink very cold water the body uses up energy to heat it up as it filters through and, as water is calorie-free, this, in theory, gives you 'negative calories'. However, as one scientist estimates, you would need to drink about 1.2 litres (2 pints) of very cold water to 'cancel out' the calories in one small digestive biscuit (although he admitted he could be wrong!).

Foods promoted as having 'negative calories' are those which are naturally very low in calories anyway – e.g. celery and cabbage. These do use up energy in their digestion and, certainly, a diet high in them will help control weight, if they are eaten instead of higher-calorie foods. Indeed, at around 7 calories per 100g, leafy vegetables may, after accounting for dietary-induced thermogenesis (see 'Calories don't count', p. 70), provide the body with no more than a calorie or two. But there is no proper research to show exactly what percentage of the total calories in celery and other vegetables is burnt in the digestive process, so this is simply speculation.

But man (and woman) cannot live on celery alone, and foods that are high in protein (see Chapter Five) which cause the body's metabolic rate to speed up the most are the most useful in achieving and maintaining weight loss.

False: a low-fat diet is the best way to slim

The low-fat diet was perhaps the biggest star of all, in terms of diets, throughout all the years I edited *Slimmer* magazine in the 1970s and '80s, and, indeed, for most of the years since. The biggest diet books of those days – *The Hip and Thigh Diet* and *The F-Plan*, among others – were all low-fat-based, even if dressed up in various guises.

Even today, the low-fat message is still around, and one that most people continue to believe is the healthiest way to control weight.

✱ *The truth*

There is mounting evidence to suggest that a reasonable amount of fat in the diet, rather than the low – 20 per cent or less – levels of low-fat diets, can actually help weight loss. And there is also growing research on the theory that low-fat diets can, in fact, hinder weight loss.

For example, several different research projects show that nuts (one of the highest-fat foods you can find) are linked with successful weight loss, for reasons which we will explore further in Chapter Five. Nuts contain unsaturated fats – and the health benefits of a reasonable amount of these fats (found also in seeds and various plant-based oils in our diets) are very important.

Australian research into overweight exercisers found that the group who had a regular intake of the omega-3 fats (found, for example, in oily fish) lost considerably more weight than the other groups studied under similar conditions. And several studies show that greater improvements in waist circumference, body-fat composition and blood-glucose levels occur when a high-carb, low-fat diet is replaced with a higher-fat, higher-protein diet.

Fat also creates satiety – much more, for instance, than carbohydrates. Low-fat manufactured foods, produced especially for people watching their weight, may contain just as many calories as higher-fat equivalents because they contain more sugars. They may also induce people to eat more, and this could be because they don't satisfy hunger.

False: you must drink eight glasses of water a day

People seem to get very confused over the issue of water – how much to drink, when to drink, what type. Rumours fly around and I get countless emails asking: 'Is it true if you drink water with a meal, the food won't digest and turns to fat?'; 'Is it true you need 4–5 litres (7–9 pints) of water a day for proper hydration?'; 'Does drinking water bloat you?'; 'Does water help you detox?'. And so on.

✱ *The truth*
Water is a calorie-free drink. I would call it natural, which it can be – but, of course, nearly all of the water we drink has been through processing and/or recycling, so it's not exactly natural. But it's the nearest thing we've got to a pure drink.

So what is a good amount of water to drink? The standard classic formula, first produced by the US National Academy of Sciences (NAS), is that an average adult needs around 1ml (0.035fl oz) of fluid a day for each calorie that he or she burns. So for an average person consuming 2000 calories that is 2 litres (3½ pints) a day, which equates to about eight 250ml (9fl oz) glasses. On that basis, obese people consuming, say, 3000 calories a day, would then need 3 litres (6.3 pints), and so on.

However, this formula relates to your entire fluid intake during the course of the day, not just water. It includes the water content of foods and drinks other than water. The NAS explained that much of the body's daily fluid needs could be met via the fluid content of food alone.

There may be times – such as when you take a lot of exercise, are ill, out in hot, dry weather, have eaten a lot of salty food – when you may need more liquids than normal. Thirst is not always a reliable indicator for dehydration; sometimes the thirst signal (especially in people who are not used to reading their body signals, which applies to many overweight people) doesn't come through strongly or quickly enough. Mostly, you won't die or even faint through short-term dehydration but you need to use common sense. The best test for whether you are getting enough fluids is to take a look at your urine – if it is a very pale colour, you are hydrated. The darker it gets, the more dehydrated you are. Aim to keep it pale with just a hint of light straw. Also, think about how often you go to the loo – if you're going fewer than four times a day, you may not be drinking enough.

I am not sure where the 'don't drink with meals' idea started, but sipping water with a meal will not do you harm, nor will it increase your weight or hamper digestion. After all, all food contains water – some fruits and vegetables are almost all water and they are the very foods often cited as being the best for weight loss. Your stomach doesn't really know whether the water that just arrived in it is part of a piece of fruit or whether you sipped it separately. I believe that the idea behind this myth is that water dilutes the stomach acids too much and thus you won't be able to begin the process of food breakdown and digestion. I can't find any science to back that up when water is consumed in normal quantities.

As for bloating, well carbonated drinks can cause gas in the intestines which may bloat, so people prone to gas might prefer to choose still water. However, unless you drink a great deal of water in a short space of time, the body can process what you drink and excrete it as urine – it doesn't hang around at belly level, bloating you out.

It's all about common sense. There have been cases where people died from drinking too much water in too short a time (e.g. several litres in less than half an hour) because the kidneys couldn't process the water quickly enough, resulting in too low a concentration of sodium in the blood leading to swelling of the brain. But this is very rare.

So now to the nitty gritty: can a certain amount of water help you to lose weight or stay on a diet? Much was made in 2009 of research on rats which seemed to show that well-hydrated rats were thinner than other rats, and that they might be more able to metabolise fat and glucose in their bodies. However, this was tenuous research in early stages, conducted on rats and not humans. Another study in 2003 found that metabolic rate increases by up to 30 per cent, following water consumption and is sustained for over an hour. This was thought partly to be due to the energy needed to heat the water. However, the long-term effect of increased water consumption and weight loss has not been studied, so more work needs to be done. There is also evidence to show that proper hydration improves performance during exercise – in resistance (strength) training, for example.

However, a recent review of all the studies done on water and health found little evidence that consuming more than you need for average hydration has any benefits to health.

Meanwhile, the facts remain that water is calorie-free and one of the cheapest and least controversial drinks. Some people say that drinking a glass of water fifteen minutes or so before a meal helps them to feel full and thus eat less at the meal, so it may be a useful tool for slimmers (though there is no scientific research that this will work).

So in conclusion, the eight glasses of water a day theory may be not far off the mark as a way of helping you to lose weight, even if there is little science behind it. It is certainly much better to drink water than to consume sugary, high-calorie drinks, such as colas, cordials and so on, or even fruit juice; and I believe it is also much better to drink water than artificially sweetened low-calorie drinks (of which more in the slimmer's foods section, see below and in Chapter Five). But note that tea – black, green, white and herbal – is good too, and even coffee (which speeds metabolism) and beer have their place. Water is not the only drink.

False: high-protein diets are dangerous

Dr Atkins gave protein a bad name. His early diet books and programmes, focusing on cutting out almost all carbs (e.g. fruit and vegetables, as well as grains and other starches) and eating a diet truly rich in animal protein (and also in animal and dairy fat), got a lot of stick from many sides of the medical profession and from nutritionists and the health media, myself included. It was felt that diets so high in saturated fats were unhealthy and would put people at risk of damaging their health and even early death.

✴ *The truth*
While few health professionals today would recommend the original Atkins diet, very many do support the idea that a high-protein diet can help people lose weight and keep it off. The difference is that today the protein is likely to be either lean animal protein – i.e. where the saturated-fat content is kept low – or from plant sources, such as nuts, seeds and pulses, which, almost all nutrition experts agree, are indeed truly healthy foods.

A diet that is reasonably high in healthy proteins has been shown, time and again, to speed metabolism, help satiety, blood-sugar levels (e.g. in people with insulin resistance and diabetes) and to help reduce a fat belly and visceral fat (that packed inside the body around the organs).

So a high-protein diet isn't dangerous – it's all about the actual type of protein you eat, how much and what else you eat besides. I tend to favour a 30:30:40 ratio; that is, 30 per cent each of protein and fat and 40 per cent of carbohydrates. This does somewhat go against the recommendations of several official bodies which quote at least 50 per cent carbohydrates for a healthy diet, but more on that in Chapter Five.

False: special slimmers' foods will help me lose weight

Billions of pounds' worth of special 'diet' foods have been sold to would-be slimmers over the past decades. The supermarkets are still full of 'low-fat', 'low-calorie', 'low-sugar' and 'light' options, aimed at people who are worried about their weight. They are promoted as a healthy way to help people reduce their calorie intake. There are also special slimmers' bars, shakes, soups and ready-meal ranges, some of which are even promoted in pharmacies and, of course on the internet.

✱ *The truth*

If they work – why are we collectively getting fatter? As *the Consumers' Association* found, these products tend to cost more than other foods, so it is likely that it is the retailers, as usual, who get fatter while we don't get thinner! They also found that many foods marketed as aids to slimming are, in fact, no lower in calories/fat/sugar than other products that are not marketed as such.

A lot of 'slimming' foods are misleading. For example, many are lower in calories simply because they are smaller. A typical 'non-guilt' bar with cereal/chocolate, for example, may weigh only 20–25g (¾–1oz), compared with an 'ordinary' one that may weigh 40–50g (1½–2oz), but you pay the same money, or even more, for the smaller bar. Similarly, slimming breads are, per slice, smaller and lighter. Also, many slimmer's complete ready meals manage to reduce the calories by making the servings small, so many people are left feeling hungry with more temptation to snack afterwards.

And 'light' versions of high-cal, high-fat foods are often just marginally lower in calories than their normal counterparts. Others, while reducing fat, may add more sugar. Many low-fat fruit yogurts, for example (often considered by dieters to be an ideal dessert), are high in sugar.

But it seems that we are beginning to work all this out for ourselves. A Mintel report found that sales of 'diet' foods have levelled off in the last few years, prompting manufacturers to come up with new ways to reel us in.

Aside from the practical reasons why special slimmers' foods may not be such a good idea, however, research proves what we knew anyway – that they don't actually help you to eat less. One 2008 research paper from Duke University, USA, found that rats fed artificial sweetener actually put on more weight than the control rats, while another study found that rats given sweetener ate more afterwards. As I explained earlier, animal experiment results may not transfer to humans, but there is evidence that some types of sweetener – aspartame has been cited – actually stimulate the appetite, thus cancelling out any low-calorie benefits. And human studies show that if we feel we have been 'good' by eating special low-calorie foods and meals, we tend to eat more after to reward ourselves.

False: sugar is needed for energy

Many a chocolate bar or bag of sweets has been sold to someone who believes they need the 'hit' of energy that it will give them. They may be feeling a bit light-headed, weak or tired, having sat at their desk for three hours with nothing to eat. Or they may have been wandering around the shopping centre for a while and suddenly been overwhelmed by the urge for something sweet. 'My blood sugars are low,' they'll say. 'I have to have a Mars bar!'

✱ The truth

Heavily refined and processed carbohydrates, such as snack foods high in simple sugars – often fructose, in the form of corn syrup, which may be even worse than sucrose (see p. 84) – do give a quick boost to blood-sugar levels. The sugars are the only nutrients apart from alcohol and water-soluble vitamins and minerals that can pass directly from the stomach into the bloodstream. Other starches, fats and proteins cannot do this. And this 'quick energy' is probably responsible for the myth that we actually need sugar for energy.

But we don't. Our bodies can convert starches, fats and proteins into usable energy and these types of food also provide a range of other important nutrients, such as vitamins, minerals, fibre, essential fats, plant chemicals and so on. We could happily live without sugar, sweets, sugary 'energy' drinks and so on. There may be certain occasions for certain people when a hit of instant sugar is needed – for diabetics, perhaps, for high-level sportspeople and so on (who should both be advised by professionals on their correct nutrition, in any case). But for most of us, in normal circumstances, we would be much better off eating small, regular meals containing a mix of protein, fat and low-GI carbs to stave off the symptoms of low blood sugar. These are the foods that keep the level stable, for the very reason that they *do* take longer to be broken down and absorbed into the bloodstream.

Indeed, regular snacking on high-sugar foods or drinks (and this includes fructose – see p. 60 – and glucose) can have both short- and long-term detrimental side effects. In the short term, the sugary snack or drink promotes the quick release of insulin from the pancreas to deal with the sugars hitting the blood and remove them for use in the cells. Once the insulin has done its job the blood-sugar levels will become low again – leaving you, possibly, wanting yet another sugar hit. In the long term, if you repeat this pattern regularly and eat a lot of sugary foods, your body may become 'insulin resistant'. This is a pre-diabetic state in which your body's response to insulin becomes blunted, so that the pancreas needs to produce more and more insulin to counter the effects of the sugar and, eventually, cannot cope. While other factors can also contribute to insulin resistance (overeating in general and eating too many other types of carbohydrate can also promote high blood-sugar levels, for example), sugar is a nutrient-devoid, high-calorie simple carb that you'd do well to avoid when you can.

So next time you consider reaching for the sweet snack between meals – think again. (See Chapter Five for information about healthier snacks and drinks.)

False: calories don't count

Many people – celebrities are particularly guilty of this – believe that weight loss and control is all about the type of food that you eat, rather than the actual calorie content of your diet. Therefore, certain foods, or even whole food groups, are avoided, while others are eaten to excess.

✱ The truth
Research from Harvard University, financed by the US National Institutes of Health and published in 2009, seems to prove that reducing calories in the diet to a sufficient level to produce an energy deficit, rather than the type of diet you follow, is the key to weight loss: 'It comes down to how much you put in your mouth – it's not a question of eating a particular type of diet,' said Frank Sacks, one of the lead researchers.

That said, there is a body of interesting research that shows our long-term ways of measuring the number of calories in what we eat can be flawed. Calorie

---

WHAT IS DIETARY-INDUCED THERMOGENESIS (DIT)?

Our bodies 'burn off' what we consume in three ways:

- by just existing (our 'basal metabolic rate' or resting metabolic rate, which accounts for about 60 per cent of total energy expenditure).
- by activity (moving or exercising, for example, which accounts for about 30 per cent of total energy expenditure).
- through dietary-induced thermogenesis or DIT, which is the energy used in processing and using food/drink, and which accounts on average for about 10 per cent of total energy expenditure.

Depending on what you eat and drink, the figure can fall or rise considerably, but by increasing your body's DIT, you can help it to lose weight and/or maintain a good weight.

content on packaging is usually measured by subjecting the food to a calorimeter – it burns the food and the amount of energy created is measured. But humans don't burn food in the same way as a calorimeter, and it's been found that various factors will influence the actual and precise calorie content of what you eat, usually by affecting dietary induced thermogenesis (DIT).

DIT accounts for between 3 and 30 per cent of our total energy expenditure. Here are some of the factors which can affect it:

- The consistency of food – soft foods use less energy to digest than hard ones.
- The state of food – cooked food uses less energy to digest than raw.
- Finely chopped food, such as minced meat, uses less energy to digest than bigger pieces of food, such as a steak (because chewing uses energy).
- Low-fibre foods use less energy to digest than high-fibre ones.

Having said that, at the time of writing, the calorie content guidelines printed on food packets and published in books such as the official *Manual of Nutrition* (the one I use) are still a good guide to the amount of calories you're eating, and until we have a better method, they can be helpful.

There is also some truth in the idea that certain foods are better than others at aiding slimming and weight maintenance. Studies show that some types of foods are more satisfying than others as they help you feel full for longer – high-protein foods are particularly good, and low-GI foods, and fat, for example. However, the baseline is that if you eat too much of these types of foods, you could still get fatter or fail to lose weight.

And foods that may hinder weight loss could perhaps include simple carbohydrates which can have a poor effect on blood-sugar levels and may increase cravings, hunger and even cause insulin resistance.

The key to your own personal success may be in finding your own best foods and ways to make sure that the calorie deficit happens.

Body and Lifestyle: Myths and Truths

Usually false: my slow metabolism is keeping me fat

Overweight and obese people often believe that they have a slow metabolic rate which means they can't lose weight. They say things like, 'I eat like a mouse and am still fat' or, 'I hardly eat a thing, honestly'.

* *The truth*

Although certain medical conditions – such as hypothyroidism (underactive thyroid gland, see below) and some medications – e.g. certain anti-depressants – can cause the metabolic rate to slow down, for most people, being overweight actually increases metabolic rate.

In fact, the fatter you are, the higher your metabolic rate is likely to be. In a simple sense, all the metabolic rate measures is the amount of calories that you use up in living – in maintaining your body, moving around, repairing it and so on. So the heavier you are, the more calories you will need in order to do all of that. Think of shopping. You find it harder to lug two heavy sacks of potatoes home than you do one small bag – it takes more energy to get the heavy items home. Similarly, it takes more energy to lug a larger body home than it does a smaller one. This principle is also behind the fact that when people try to lose weight, they find a lot goes off in the early stages and, as they get slimmer, they find it harder to shift the final pounds: the slimmer you get, the lower your metabolic rate gets (all other factors being equal).

So if you are overweight and about to embark on a slimming campaign – be grateful while you can for your fat, which will result in good weight loss in the immediate future!

Lastly – research shows that obese people underestimate their calorie intake by an average of 40 per cent – sometimes, by as much as 800 calories a day.

Probably false: it's my glands

This is a vague allusion to the thyroid gland, which is the gland most often thought of as controlling weight. However, it is rarely the case.

* *The truth*

The thyroid gland, at the base of the front of the neck, helps regulate the body's metabolism and, if it is malfunctioning, can be a cause of weight gain. However, it is estimated that only 3 per cent of cases of obesity are caused by an underactive thyroid. This diagnosis is more likely if you also suffer from unexplained tiredness, coldness, dry skin and constipation.

If you think you have thyroid problems, go and see your GP. If he or she decides to test you and you come out negative, then I am afraid if any glands at all are at fault, it's your saliva glands. The good news is that they can still be satisfied by great-tasting food, even when you choose to lose weight.

Unlikely: I'm not fat, I just have big/heavy bones

This is another great excuse – often used, no doubt, because no one in the room can really readily prove or disprove it.

✱ *The truth*

Human bone doesn't weigh that much – compared with, say, a piece of metal or wood. That is because it contains around 50 per cent water and air. In people of average weight, the skeleton forms just a small percentage of their total weight – around 15 per cent in men and just 12 per cent in women. Also, healthy young adults will not vary that much in the amount of bone they carry. Yes, build does vary – but just because you may have, say, bigger hip bones than someone else or a broader back, that doesn't mean you have to carry extra fat as well.

One thing is for sure – if, over your adult years, you have put on weight, it certainly isn't extra bone weight. Your bone mass is fixed by the time you are in your early thirties, after which you can't add to it, but it will slowly diminish (or rapidly in some cases, after the menopause). The extra weight will be fat and/or muscle (more likely fat, unless you have taken up weight-lifting on a regular basis or similar).

Possible: it's my hormones

Although it is easy to use 'hormones' as an excuse to overeat, there is something in the idea that your hormones affect hunger, appetite, weight and shape.

✱ *The truth*

Hormones are chemicals which help to co-ordinate, balance and regulate processes in the body. There are different types of hormones – for example, growth hormones, sex hormones, stress hormones, such as adrenaline and others. Insulin is a hormone, and as we've already seen (see p. 69), insulin and body weight are linked. The female hormones which produce the menstrual cycle – oestrogen and progesterone, for example – are known to have an effect on appetite, often increasing it in the premenstrual phase for many women and during pregnancy. And the steroidal hormone cortisol is produced by the adrenal gland, high levels of which are associated with abdominal fat. The complete workings of the hormones, their influence on body weight and ways in which they may be harnessed to regulate weight have yet to be completely understood.

Note: the fact that hormones are produced by various glands around the body may lend some credibility to the 'It's my glands' theory in this instance.

Possible: I'm not tall enough

I have a friend who is five foot tall and struggles with her weight. 'If I were five foot, seven,' she says, 'I would be really thin!' It's supposed to be a joke, but there is some truth behind it.

✳ *The truth*

If you are shorter than average, you need to eat fewer calories than someone who is taller than you in order to maintain a reasonable weight. (This presupposes that all other factors are equal, such as sex, age, level of activity and so on.) This is because the smaller the animal, in general, the less food it needs to survive. Why does a mouse eat less than a cat?

That isn't to say they don't or can't put on weight – they can and do – but just as fat people have a higher metabolic rate than thin people, so tall people have a higher metabolic rate than short people.

It isn't fair, but taller people have been dealt a better hand if they want to indulge themselves and stay slim. However, I look at it another way. Think of all the money you're saving by not having to eat so much!

Possible: I'm addicted to food

People who 'crave' sugar, chocolate, or a variety of other types of foods (sometimes salty ones such as crisps, or starchy things like cake or bread) often claim they are 'addicted' to these items and can't give them up.

✳ *The truth*

While the line on this from most professionals has been that food cravings are not actual addictions, but simply 'comfort eating' or a response to other factors (see hormones above), recent research indicates a stronger than previously thought similarity between the need for food – or certain types of food – and the need for alcohol and addictive drugs.

In 2006, researchers at Brookhaven Labs in the USA found that food affects the brain's dopamine systems. This powerful neurotransmitter plays a key role in addiction – alcohol and addictive drugs disrupt the way in which it works, effectively taking away freedom of choice. Just like drug addicts, obese people compared with healthy slim people have fewer dopamine 'receptors'. The researchers also found that the more obese people are, the fewer dopamine 'receptors' they have, which may go some way towards explaining why many morbidly obese people have trouble controlling their food intake.

More recent research in New Zealand has highlighted similarities between food and drug addiction. It found that sugary foods stimulate the same areas of the brain as those involved in nicotine and alcohol addition. Sugary foods/ drinks and simple carbohydrates release serotonin, a chemical that initially improves your mood and makes you feel good. However, the effect is just temporary and can lead to a rollercoaster effect. As with drugs, addicts become tolerant and need more of their chosen substance to achieve the same effect. The lows that follow the highs may also be like those found in recognised addictions. And it's not just the physical effects that cause this – research carried out by the charity MIND found that in the long term, a diet rich in chocolate causes negative emotions and increases depression – because of the guilt eating it brings about.

Dr Robert Hill, a leading UK consultant psychologist in addictions, says:

> 'For the majority of people periodic overconsumption of food will be related to anxiety and stress, and occurs as a form of positive reward and/or as a means of controlling some part of their life when the rest of it feels out of control. This is a form of negative reinforcement (where food is used in order not to experience something unpleasant). The opposite, positive reinforcement, is when we do something for its rewarding properties in and of itself, thus the gourmet will eat for the sheer pleasure of food.'

Specific foods may have specific further effects. For example, chocolate contains not only sugar, but also relaxants and stimulants found in the cocoa bean and crisps and bread, although not sweet, are high-carbohydrate refined foods. More and more research is linking such foods with obesity.

Maybe, then, food can be truly addictive. The good news is, however, that a few simple strategies can help even the most hard-bitten addict to recover. In Chapter Ten, Dr Hill helps us to do this!

Unlikely: I'm overweight, but it's all muscle

There has been a lot of publicity in recent years about how the standard measure for testing weight – the Body Mass Index – can give false impressions. For example, top-class sportspeople can come out with a high BMI, even in the 'obese' category, because their muscle mass makes them heavy, even though they have a low body-fat percentage.

∗ The truth

However, for most of us, trying to use this excuse to explain our high BMI doesn't wash. Normal people who do a normal amount of exercise – and today in the UK, the average is less than half an hour a day – will not make sufficient lean tissue (muscle) to bulk up their bodies to such an extent. It takes a great deal of specific weight-bearing exercise, done on an almost daily basis, to achieve that.

So sadly, if you're Mr or Ms Average, and your BMI is high, you are probably carrying too much body fat.

Unlikely: it's a virus

This idea gained a lot of press coverage when, in 2007, the research doctor who had spent ten years studying a possible link between the cold virus adenovirus-36 and obesity, released the results of a study of 1000 obese patients which found that obese people were three times as likely as slim people to carry the virus.

∗ The truth

Most professionals feel the case is nowhere near proved and that if there is a link, it accounts for no more than a tiny number of the billion cases of obesity worldwide.

Maybe it is comforting to think that your fat belly isn't due to your food intake but to that cold you had a few years ago; sadly, however, that really may be wishful thinking.

Unlikely: I'm always hungry, so I must need the food

The perceived wisdom here is that if you are always eating, it must be because your body somehow needs the food. However, this is infrequently the case.

∗ The truth

Some medical conditions can cause you to feel unnaturally hungry – diabetes or a thyroid complaint, for instance. And pregnancy or, as we've seen, the premenstrual phase, can increase hunger too. If you have any other symptoms, such as extreme tiredness or weight loss you should see your GP to exclude particular conditions.

Ruling those out, however, if you're eating a lot and putting on weight, you probably don't need the amount of calories you are consuming. In today's world, where food is readily available everywhere, it is very easy to mistake simple 'seeing food and eating it' for hunger.

If you eat a diet high in 'junk food', which may be low in nutrients, such as vitamins, minerals and essential fats, for example, your body will be getting the calories but will still need better nutrition. However, there is little, if any, evidence to show that the body recognises when you are low on a particular nutrient and sends you a message to eat.

(For detailed information on the thorny subject of hunger and how to deal with it, see Chapters Five and Ten.)

Possible: I'm fat because I'm depressed

With overweight and depression, it is sometimes hard to know which came first. Are you feeling depressed because you are fat, or are you indulging in too much comfort eating because you are depressed?

✱ The truth

Well, the jury is still out, but there has been some interesting recent research from Rush University in the USA showing that depression and central body fat (the fat around and within the abdomen) are linked. The study's lead researcher believes that depression may trigger the accumulation of this fat by means of certain chemical changes – perhaps the production of cortisol (see p. 73).

It is certainly true that 'fat and happy' is a myth, or a rarity at best. Population studies show that obese people are infrequently genuinely happy with their size or life and the jolly front (if there is one) is just that – a front. The US National Institute of Mental Health looked at 9000 people and found that obesity was associated with a 25 per cent increase in the incidence of depression and mental disorders.

The problem is that depression, by definition, inhibits the will to 'do', which often includes the changes necessary to lose weight. If the cycle of eating–overweight–depression, followed by more eating–more overweight–more depression can be penetrated, the pattern can be broken. Any kind of activity is a great way to do this as physical activity is strongly linked both with beating depression and with weight control.

Possible: it's my genes

Blaming our genes for being overweight – or indeed, too thin – is natural. After all, we inherit our eye colour, our looks and our build from our parents and previous generations, so why not our propensity or otherwise to put on weight?

* *The truth*

According to the *International Journal of Obesity*, 127 different genes have been linked to some aspect of obesity. Genes appear to contribute to obesity in various ways. For example, they may 'pass on' down the generations a slow metabolism, a tendency to overeat or to be physically inactive, an impaired ability to burn calories from fat and/or a tendency to have a higher number of body-fat cells than average and a tendency to store body fat.

The message is that if one or both of your parents are significantly overweight, you're much more likely to become obese than if your parents are normal weight. But the strength of the genetic influence on weight varies quite a bit from person to person and physical activity can blunt these genetic effects. Indeed, the results of a large study of Amish people published in 2008 show that the most active of these people overrode any genetic tendency to obesity.

Often true: I put on weight because I gave up smoking

Nicotine speeds up the metabolic rate, dulls the appetite and gives the mouth and hands something to do, other than eating – three reasons why smokers, on average, weigh less than non-smokers.

* *The truth*

About 80 per cent of people who give up smoking put on weight (about 3.2kg/ 7lb, on average). Of these, according to the UK Government, 'most' lose some or all of that weight over time.

Two factors are worth mentioning here: if, as a smoker, you were slim or thin, as many are, then you can afford to put on a little weight without becoming fat. It may even be a good thing (for more about ideal weight, see Chapter Three). Also, if you stop smoking, your lungs will be free from tobacco pollution and you should find it easier and more pleasurable to take up regular exercise. Indeed, research shows that exercise is one of the keys to keeping away from the cigarettes – perhaps because it acts as a natural 'high', can reduce stress and induce relaxation and better sleep.

A grain of truth: I sleep more than most people, so I put on weight

It seems reasonable to suppose that if you spend long hours in bed, you will use up less energy during your life than someone who sleeps less and is more active.

* *The truth*

Research on the human metabolic rate over many years has produced average figures for the amount of calories we burn up at rest, work and play. An average-sized woman (say, 63.5kg/10 stone) will burn approximately 60 calories per hour when her body is 'at rest'. In waking hours, if that woman is physically active, she may burn up on average throughout the day another 30 calories per hour. So if she is in bed for eight hours, that is 480 calories burnt. And for the remaining sixteen hours, she burns (16 x 90) 1440 calories, making a total of 1920.

If the same woman stayed in bed for eleven hours, that would only reduce her daily calorie burn to 1830. The difference of 90 calories of unused energy per day would account for no more than about 90g (3oz) weight gain a week, all other factors being equal.

However, research shows that many of us today are not that physically active. A sedentary job and evenings spent watching TV may mean we burn only an extra 10 per cent of calories over and above our resting metabolic rate (RMR) during the day – i.e. 66 calories an hour when we are not sleeping. That would mean burning 1536 calories in twenty-four hours if you slept eight hours a night, or 1518 calories if you sleep eleven hours a night – a difference of just 18 calories a day.

So for the purposes of burning calories, it would seem that it is more important to be active during the hours you are out of bed, rather than worrying too much about how many hours you spend in bed.

However, it's not that simple. It doesn't mean that if seven to eight hours' sleep is good, four to five hours is better, in terms of weight control. There is quite a bit of research from the USA and Canada which appears to show that both short sleep duration (fewer than five hours a night), as well as long sleep duration (more than nine hours a night) are linked in some more fundamental way with obesity, diabetes and other health problems. Indeed, one study found that obesity was more likely in short sleepers than in long sleepers – perhaps because getting less sleep might disrupt natural hormonal balances, thus reducing the amount of leptin, a hormone which controls appetite.

Stress may also be a factor in both reducing the length and quality of sleep and increasing eating and other behaviour that may result in weight gain.

More research needs to be done, but meanwhile, it is still the 'average' sleeper who has the best chance of being slim with seven to eight hours' sleep a night being the right amount to help prevent obesity.

Unlikely: eating late at night means you don't burn up the calories

Following on from the 'no carbs in the evening' theory (see p. 58), it is often said that the later you eat, the more calories from that meal are laid down as fat because while you sleep, you aren't burning them off.

✱ *The truth*

The 'sleep' question that we just discussed shows that many people hardly burn more calories during the day than they do when they are asleep, which knocks this theory on the head straight away.

In addition, the process of digesting and utilising food (or storing the surplus as fat) is more complex than the picture described. Even if the digestion and sorting process is complete before you wake in the morning and any surplus carbs, fat or protein have been suitably stored in their correct places in the body – even as body fat – the human body is cleverly designed to compensate over the course of days, or weeks, to release that energy from food as and when you need it. This means that you don't need to worry all that much about precisely how much you eat at each meal, or even each day, or at what time you eat, as long as your overall calorie input – calorie output balance is maintained over time.

The only downside about eating late at night is it may give some people indigestion and wakefulness. On the other hand, not eating in the evening can cause wakefulness too, as it results in low blood-sugar levels, which can disrupt sleep.

False: it's lack of exercise, not too much food, that makes me put on weight

There have been some research studies – often funded by food companies (!!) that appear to show that weight gain is down not to eating too much, but simply to a lack of exercise.

✱ *The truth*

This is an extremely simplistic view of the obesity problem. For most people it is a combination of both overeating and not enough exercise. Research on the eating habits and energy expenditure of US citizens published by the European Association for the Study of Obesity in 2009 found that the rise in obesity in the States since the 1970s is almost all down to eating more, rather than exercising less. On the other hand, a large study published in the *International Journal of*

Obesity in 2009, based on the citizens of nine European countries, found that physical activity is inversely associated with both BMI and waist circumference – i.e. the less exercise you do, the fatter you are.

There are more studies on this subject, and the overall conclusion I draw is the obvious: in most people, obesity is a result of both eating too much (for their own needs) and of not being active enough. If you are overweight and want to continue eating the amount you are eating, the only way to lose weight is to do lots of exercise. But if you eat less, you can lose weight without much extra exercise at all.

You should also bear in mind that it does take a lot of exercise to produce a measurable weight loss. As a rule of thumb, an hour's brisk walking every day for a week would burn up an extra 2000 or so calories (over your RMR) which in theory would help you to lose about 225g (8oz). Assuming the extra exercise doesn't make you hungry, so you eat more.

That said, exercise is a health-promoting activity vital for human wellbeing, and there is very good evidence that *maintaining* weight loss over time is all about regular exercise (for more on this, see Chapter Nine).

In conclusion, what does all this really tell us about ourselves? We are sometimes gullible, we can be masters at kidding ourselves, and that most of us are in desperate need of some lessons in body intelligence – the first step of which is, as we've seen, knowledge.

The next chapter will set out the facts rather than the fiction about food, health, weight and your body. This is where your escape from the fat trap begins to become reality.

5
Food for Thought

This chapter is the 'knowledge' corner. It explains what is most likely to help you succeed, by setting out the facts about food and health, and the type of diet that allows your body to look after itself.

One-minute Nutrition Course

You may think of this as the 'boring bit' if you like, but I think it's important to do a quick recap of what the human body needs to keep itself in good running order:

Macronutrients (ingested in large quantities) are carbohydrates (subdivided into starches and sugars), protein and fat (and perhaps also alcohol, although alcohol isn't a *necessary* macronutrient, just one that many of us do consume).

All these provide energy (kilocalories, often termed calories) to keep us alive. Carbohydrates have nearly 4 calories per gram, protein has 4 calories per gram and fat 9. Alcohol has 5. (Note: figures are approximate.)

Then we have the micronutrients (needed in small or very small quantities), which are vitamins, minerals and the relatively new boys on the block – all the other chemicals which have been discovered in our foods, often umbrella-termed as phytochemicals/antioxidants.

We also need water, without which we can't survive more than a short time (although much of the water we do need to survive can be provided by food; many food types contain 50–90 per cent water by weight and some are over 95 per cent water). And we need what is commonly known as dietary fibre – loosely grouped into insoluble fibre (the parts of the food that we eat that remain largely undigested and pass out in the faeces) and soluble fibre, although there are other types of fibre-like compounds in food.

Everything that we eat consists of one or more (usually more) of the above. Cheddar cheese, for example, is a mix of fat and protein, potatoes are a mix of carbs and protein with a dot of fat (although refined white sugar and highly refined vegetable oils contain very little besides sucrose and fat, respectively).

End of one-minute nutrition course!

The Mystery of the 'Balanced Diet'

For decades there has been hot debate about just what are the right proportions of all the above to produce the 'best' diet for health and weight maintenance. Sometimes, it seems that no two professionals can agree, although for a time it seemed that a 'low-fat, high-carb diet' was proclaimed by most experts to be the best, and thus the huge low-fat food industry was born. At the same time, the (in)famous Dr Robert Atkins, over in the USA, was persuading those of us who were not following a low-fat diet to choose the very high-protein diet that he promoted – an idea that most professionals scorned.

Um – but now, well, we're not so sure. In fact, Dr Atkins could have been more right than we suspected. So here I want to explain what does seem to be certain about the right balance of nutrients.

Note: it's important to know that the advice I give here (and my reporting of the advice from scientists across the world) is intended for adults in normal health. If you have any specific health problems, allergies etc. for which you are receiving medical advice, I would always urge you to ask for more personal recommendations about your diet – your own doctor should refer you to a dietician for whatever help you need.

Carbohydrates – good (well, mostly) in moderation

The main purpose of high-carbohydrate foods is to provide you with energy to power, maintain and repair your body. While fat, alcohol and protein can also provide your body with energy (calories), carbs are the most easily utilised source, and unlike protein and fat, they serve no other purpose, as they can't repair, or make, lean tissue, such as muscle. If you eat more carbohydrate than you require for energy, the surplus is either stored in the muscles or liver, or converted to body fat.

FACT

If you were to eat nothing but pure carbohydrate, you would become progressively weaker, as your body would break down your lean tissue in order to provide your vital organs (the heart, lungs and brain) with the amino acids and other substances they need to keep functioning. However much carb you ate, this would still happen. You could even put on weight, as all the surplus carbs unused for energy would convert to body fat – but you would, eventually, die.

Most of us know by now that there are 'good' carbs and 'bad' carbs. Starches tend to be branded the goodies, sugars the baddies.

✱ Starches

Starchy foods are plant-based (there are no carbs in meat or fish). High-starch foods include cereals, most pulses and many root vegetables. If these foods are left 'whole' – i.e. they are not put through much in the way of processing – they are likely to contain high levels of dietary fibre, mostly the insoluble type. They will also be a good, even rich, source of a variety of vitamins, minerals and plant chemicals, and many are low-GI foods (see box, p. 86). If they are highly refined (e.g. white bread, refined breakfast cereals, white rice) their fibre and micronutrient content is reduced (but in the UK white bread has to be fortified with vitamins and minerals to replace those lost) and their GI level is likely to be high.

✱ Sugars

Sugars are sweet carbs found in natural foods, in greatest quantity in fruit. Some vegetables (e.g. carrots) contain reasonable amounts of sugars too.

WHAT YOU NEED TO KNOW ABOUT SUGAR

Research at Cambridge University has found, using new accurate sugar/urine testing equipment devised by the Medical Research Council, that we do, in fact, eat a lot more sugar than we think we do; and that obese people eat more sugary foods than non-obese people.

There has been much debate about what types of sugar have the most adverse effects on our bodies and weight. The huge rise in the USA (and, to a lesser degree, in the UK) in the use of corn syrup – a mix of fructose and glucose similar in composition to table sugar – in manufactured foods and soft drinks since the 1970s almost directly parallels the rise in obesity. (It now accounts for 10 per cent of an average US citizen's calorie intake.) Fructose, too, has come under suspicion of causing obesity after a recent trial found it tended to increase both intra-abdominal fat and insulin resistance more than did glucose. However, the same trial found that people having a high-sugar diet put on weight whether the main sugar was fructose or glucose.

At the time of writing, most nutritional scientists who have studied this thorny subject agree that much more research needs to be done, but that meanwhile, the advice to watch our total sugar intake closely for both health and weight control makes sense.

Sugars in food are often a mix of glucose and fructose. Honey is an example. Lactose is a type of sugar found in milk and dairy produce. Sugars that are naturally found in produce are termed 'intrinsic' sugars, and in the nutrition world are regarded as 'healthy', while sugar added to food during the manufacturing process (e.g. in soft drinks, cakes, biscuits, desserts, sweets, chocolate) is called 'extrinsic' sugar and is regarded as much less healthy.

Extrinsic sugars tend to have a rapid effect on blood-sugar levels and on insulin production and some intrinsic sugars can do so too. Also, some starchy carbs with a high GI are rapidly converted to blood sugar as well.

Most sugars contain no nutrients (or virtually none) other than calories and, for that reason alone, sugars should be the first candidate to be cut or reduced in your diet. For more on sugars, see box, p. 84.

✱ *How much carbohydrate?*
Official advice is that 50 per cent of your calorie intake should come from carbohydrates. For most of us, around 55 per cent of our diet is made up of carbs, but that will include sweet snacks, highly refined cereals, baked goods, packet foods, pastries, crisps and so on – and these are the things we need to cut right down on. What we should be doing is eating more 'natural', 'good' carbs – whole, unadulterated (or only somewhat adulterated, as in the rolling of oats or the husking of rice), cooked in simple ways. By cutting out a lot of the rubbish carbs from our diets, we could lose weight and reduce our total saturated and trans fat intake at the same time. So it isn't so much a question of how much, but the type of carbohydrate we eat.

✱ *The importance of the glycaemic index [GI]*
The GI – a measure of how quickly or slowly carbohydrate foods are absorbed into the bloodstream – was originally produced to help diabetics control their blood-sugar levels. A diet that contains most of its carbs in low-GI form can help protect you from insulin resistance, diabetes and heart disease and has been found to be a valuable tool for weight loss and weight loss maintenance, as it helps prevent hunger.

FACT
Vinegar and lemon juice both slow down carb absorption by up to 50 per cent. So if you do find yourself with a high-GI food, add either of these to reduce its fast effects on your blood-sugar level.

By choosing your carbs from the lower to medium end of the GI scale you will be choosing, mostly at least, the 'good carbs'.

The foods that tend to be lower on the GI are those that take longer for the body to digest. This often equates with high-fibre carbs, such as wholegrains and pulses, and/or with foods that are harder to chew, such as wholegrain bread, rather than plain wholemeal bread. Foods that tend to be high on the GI are highly processed and refined carbs, such as cornflakes and white bread. Glucose itself, pure sugar, rates 100 per cent on the index – the highest GI food of all.

Some unexpected carbs are high GI – for instance, mashed and baked potatoes are high, while new potatoes and sweet potatoes are much lower. Even different types of potato have different GI ratings (for example, King Edwards are high, while Estimas are medium). Apples are low GI, while pineapples are high. The chart below gives low, medium and high values.

However, both fat and protein eaten at the same time will help to slow down the rate of absorption of whatever carb you eat.

A ROUGH GUIDE TO THE GLYCAEMIC INDEX
Low-GI foods
- All pulses, such as lentils, chickpeas, baked beans
- Apples, peaches, grapefruit, plums, cherries, dried apricots
- Most green vegetables, mushrooms
- Natural yogurt, milk

Medium–low-GI foods
- Sweet potatoes, boiled new potatoes, sweetcorn, peas
- Pasta, oats, wholegrain breads, rye bread, pitta bread, bulgur, rice
- Grapes, oranges, kiwi, mangoes, beetroot, dates, figs

High-GI foods
- Glucose, sugar, honey
- Pineapples, bananas, raisins, melon
- Baked and mashed potatoes, parsnips, squash
- Crispbreads, wholemeal and white bread, couscous
- Cornflakes, bran flakes, instant oat cereal, puffed cereal, popcorn, crumpets

(See Further Help, p. 218, for details of where to find more information on the GI.)

Proteins - the slimline tonic of the food world

Protein is needed to build and maintain lean tissue (muscles, including the heart) and for a variety of other jobs which can't be done by either carbs or fat. Protein is made up of twenty-two amino acids, and different types of protein food provide different mixes of these, so a mix of lean animal protein, plant protein and dairy protein may be a good idea.

Protein-rich meats, poultry and fish also provide a good range of other important nutrients, such as iron, zinc, selenium and B vitamins. Oily fish will also give you essential omega-3 fats. Protein-rich dairy produce such as hard cheeses, milk and to a lesser extent yogurt, also provides calcium for your bones, A and B vitamins, as well as being a general health protector and, potentially, a good source of probiotics for gut health, with a capacity to help weight loss too. It has also been found that calcium can block fat absorption and can increase leptin, the hormone that helps to curb appetite, while the probiotics (micro-organisms) in yogurt seem to lessen the chances of accumulating abdominal fat, according to research presented at the 2009 European Congress on Obesity. Protein-rich eggs give you a range of vitamins and minerals. Some plants, especially pulses, and also nuts and seeds, provide protein and can also give you a range of vitamins, minerals and plant chemicals (antioxidants, for example), as well as essential fats.

There is considerable research to show that a diet reasonably high in protein can help you lose weight or maintain a sensible weight. Here's why:

- Eating protein – especially animal protein – results in a higher level of 'dietary-induced thermogenesis' (DIT, see p. 70) than carbs or fat. An overview of all the research into DIT to date found the DIT effect for protein to be 20–30 per cent (for carbs it's 5–10 per cent, fat is 0–3 per cent and alcohol 10–30 per cent). So a high-protein diet can actually burn extra calories.
- Protein is digested more slowly than carbs, so helps keep blood-sugar levels even by effectively reducing the glycaemic index of a carb food if eaten at the same time (the same is also true of fats).
- Unlike carbs, protein does not encourage the release of insulin by the pancreas.
- Although protein can be converted into body fat if we eat so much of it that it cannot all be used in other ways (e.g. to maintain muscle), the body doesn't like to convert protein to fat; it would rather use carbs.
- While high-carb meals can cause 'bloating', protein doesn't encourage fluid retention.

NUTS

Research shows that not only are nuts very good for you – with anti-heart disease properties – they may also help with weight control. It seems that the fibre in nuts may block some of the nut fat from being absorbed. Nuts also have a high satiety factor as they contain oleic acid (also found in olive oil and avocados) which diminishes hunger.

Having said all that, many protein foods are also high in fat – fatty cuts of meat, chicken with the skin on, many cheeses and full-fat milk being a few examples (which also happen to be high in saturated fat too). It makes sense mostly to choose lower-fat animal protein foods, such as lean beef, skinless chicken, venison and pork fillet, and to get more fat from plant and fish proteins, such as nuts, seeds and oily fish.

Fats – no longer the baddies if you're careful

We all need fat. Indeed, even slimmers need fat.

Doctors now know that the popular very low-fat diets of the 1980s and '90s were not as healthy as we liked to think, because they tend to lower 'good' cholesterol by at least as much as they did 'bad' cholesterol. And they tended to restrict foods that contain the essential fats – nuts, seeds, oily fish for example.

Fat is a great tool for helping satiety and, like protein, helps reduce the sharp blood-sugar spurts associated with high-GI carbs. So a high Glycaemic Index baked potato topped with a knob of butter or some grated cheese will be a low-GI meal. Its only downside is that it appears to have little thermogenic (DIT) effect when you eat it (see 'Proteins', above).

Having said that, there have been several small, but scientific, trials to show that unsaturated fats (such as those found in olive oil and walnuts) have a much higher DIT effect than saturated fats (such as cream), and the conclusion is that – especially for obese people and those with fat around their middle – unsaturated oils are worth swapping to, for their DIT bonus. One 2009 trial found DIT around 25 per cent higher with olive oil and walnuts than with high-fat dairy produce. This could be why people who eat a diet high in items such as butter, cream, ice cream and fatty pastries are more likely to be obese and/or have a high waist circumference than people who eat a high-oil Mediterranean style diet.

Saturated fat (that found in largest quantities in meats and dairy produce) is still regarded by most professionals as the 'baddy', along with hydrogenated

FIVE A DAY? WELL THAT'S WRONG FOR STARTERS ...

We all know, don't we, that we should eat five portions of fruit and vegetables a day? In fact, the latest US official health advice is that nine portions a day is optimal for maximum health protection.

Five a day was the minimum recommended by the World Health Organisation back in the early 1990s. However, much research has been done since then on the benefits of vegetables and fruits and it's been found that fruit should make up no more than half of your daily fruit and vegetable allowance for a number of reasons:

- Fruit does not give you all the beneficial plant compounds you need. Leafy greens are particularly important for cancer prevention; orange and red vegetables, likewise.
- If you get most or all of your five (or nine) as fruit, you are taking in quite a lot of sugar and carbs and more calories, than if you eat vegetables, almost all of which are low in these. (This excludes roots like potatoes, which are classed as carbohydrates and don't count as one of your daily portions, anyway.)
- Fruit sugar (fructose) isn't always saintly and by no means all fruits are low-GI, so eating them as a between-meal snack on their own will affect blood-sugar levels.
- Worst of all is taking one of your five a day as a juice 'snack' between meals. Stripped of its fibre, a piece of fruit juiced in a glass is High-GI with a capital H.

fats – which are used much less widely in processed foods now as their negative effects on health have been documented.

Fat also offers protective and wellbeing benefits. Omega 3s, found in oily fish and some plant foods, help protect your immune system, memory and brain power, and protect against major diseases, including diabetes and cardiovascular disease. Mono-unsaturated fats found in olive oil and avocados, for example, help boost HDL 'good' cholesterol and contain plant chemicals that can help minimise inflammation. The oleic acid they contain also helps prevent hunger.

Remember: plant and fish fats are good and you should include them in your diet.

Drinks – why they could be keeping you fat

Many people, particularly children, teens and young adults, consume a sizeable portion of their daily calories in the form of drinks. Most of these calories are sugar which, as we've seen, is 'empty' calories, with a strong link to obesity and diabetes (as well as tooth decay and enamel erosion, especially when drinks are sipped throughout the day).

In the USA, soft-drink consumption has trebled since the 1970s, according to new research. A 2009 study from Columbia University in New York found that youngsters up to age nineteen who drank plain water instead of soft drinks saved an average of 235 calories every day – equating to around 9kg (24lb) of fat over the course of a year.

The average American now consumes 72.5kg (160lb) of added sugars a year, much of which is in soft drinks and much of which is the ubiquitous corn syrup (see p. 84). Eleven per cent of US calorie intake is soft drinks and juices.

Research has also found that artificial sweeteners may increase appetite and do little to prevent weight gain. Indeed, research carried out by Harvard University in 2007 found that regular consumption of artificially sweetened diet drinks increased the risk of obesity and high blood pressure. There are also still question marks over the safety of some sweeteners, though the industry will deny this.

* But juice is good, though – isn't it?
Juices are hardly any better than colas or squashes as a regular drink. They are high on the glycaemic index (see p. 85 and p. 89 for more on this) and also higher in calories than you might think. Their only real benefit nutritionally is that some types (e.g. orange) contain good amounts of vitamin C (but others, such as apple juice, may contain little).

* A nice glass of milk then?
Ah! Now you may be talking. Milk is a good source of calcium, and there is quite strong evidence to support the idea that calcium intake blocks the absorption of some of the fat in our diets. Calcium supplements have a similar effect, but calcium in dairy seems to work up to 100 per cent better. Three portions of dairy a day (equivalent to about 850ml/1½ pints of milk), containing about 1000mg of calcium, which is higher than the UK/EC recommended daily allowance (RDA) but the same as the USA's RDA),helped obese people lose 10 per cent of their weight in one trial by the leading researcher into calcium, Michael Zemel and his team.

Milk also has the benefit of being a low-GI drink, and it contains protein and B vitamins. Full-fat (whole) milk is quite high in calories, fat and saturated fat though; the ideal drink is skimmed milk. Soya milk enriched with calcium for non-milk drinkers is an alternative.

✱ Or a cup of tea ...

The much-maligned, calorie-free cup of tea of the late twentieth century is now more or less a star of the health world. What a change of image! 165 million cups a day are consumed in the UK, and the good news is that our favourite, black tea, is almost as healthy as the more expensive green and white teas. They all contain polyphenols which can help prevent CVD and heart attacks.

However, there is also some good evidence to suggest that green and white teas may actually help us to lose weight (possibly by speeding up the rate at which fat is burnt). These teas contain a nutrient called epigallocatechin, which is mostly lost when 'raw' teas are processed into black tea.

Most studies show that milk added to tea doesn't spoil its healthy or slimming effects. Three spoonfuls of sugar might though.

✱ ... or coffee?

Like tea, coffee is sounding more like a health drink every year. The latest research shows it can help protect against Alzheimer's, as well as asthma attacks, certain cancers, Parkinson's disease, gallstones and diabetes. It also improves the circulation, boosts alertness and speeds up the metabolic rate, which is useful for slimmers.

As overconsumption of strong coffee is still linked with insomnia (because of the caffeine content) it is wise to avoid drinking it in the evening – and in pregnancy limit it to 3–4 medium-strength cups a day – but otherwise, it seems to have the green light now. Coffee contains virtually no calories, but obviously if you add masses of sugar, cream, syrup flavourings or chocolate, you can rack up vast amounts of calories, fat and carbs too.

✱ And water?

All the research I've amassed shows that water is the way to go if you want to lose weight (see also p. 65).

✱ Alcohol

Most of us know by now that we are 'allowed' to drink a little alcohol and that in certain circumstances, it is said, it may actually be good for us. Red wine and other dark drinks like stout contain chemicals which act as antioxidants and may help promote a healthy heart.

But all alcohol contains calories, and some types contain quite a lot of sugar. And there is even new research casting doubt on the whole 'red-wine-is-good-for-you' idea (see box, below).

As for the beer belly: the beer industry claims that any food or drink can give you a fat belly if you have too much of it (true) and there is recent research to show that while some heavy drinkers do have fat bellies, others don't. Too many calories from alcohol can put on weight, but it doesn't necessarily end up as stomach fat alone – you could put on weight all over.

The important thing to know about alcohol is that its calories can't be put to good use in the body, so must be burnt as energy. (And it contains about 7 calories per gram – so much higher than either carbohydrates or protein, but a little lower than fat.) That means that if you are eating a high-carb, high-fat diet, as well as drinking quite a bit, your body may not get the chance to use the carb and fat calories as energy so they will end up as body fat.

Alcohol also lowers your blood sugar so may make you feel more hungry. Plus, high alcohol intake also reduces self-control and can thus encourage eating with abandon – twin facts that may have disastrous consequences.

One bit of good news though, if you like a tipple, is that the DIT effect (see p. 70) of alcohol is quite high – nearly as high as that of protein. However, that doesn't really cancel out the negative effects of over-indulgence.

My advice would be to go for a glass of good-quality red wine with your evening meal, and at other times go for spirits, which contain virtually no sugar and are about 55 calories a shot, plus a soda water or water. An old-fashioned

---

THE TRUTH ABOUT ALCOHOL STUDIES?

The relationship between alcohol and human health is largely examined by what are called 'observational studies' – i.e. simplistically, based on asking people how they live and what they drink, and pairing that up with their health. The conclusion – that low-to-moderate drinking is linked with health benefits – may simply be drawn because the people who do drink in moderation live generally healthier lifestyles than either teetotallers or heavy drinkers.

There are also a lot of academic research establishments which rely on funding from drinks manufacturers; and other trials (in the case of the French wine industry, for example) are actually directly funded by the industry, all of which has the potential to be a problem.

Before the real truth can be established, proper scientific 'randomised controlled' clinical trials need to be done.

glass of dry sherry is another option – at only about 58 calories for a good 50ml (2fl oz) shot, it is also low in sugar and even contains some minerals, such as magnesium and calcium (as do all wines). Avoid sweet wines and port as regular tipples – not only are they high in alcohol, but in sugar too. Ciders and beers are also moderate to high in sugars. All these will play havoc with your blood sugar levels, especially if you drink on an 'empty stomach'.

In conclusion I believe that if you feed yourself well – in the sense that you give your body good, nutritious food in sensible balance – then you will find the whole process of becoming a healthy weight and keeping that way, much easier to achieve.

I also strongly believe that food should be enjoyed, relished, taken time and care over. A mistake many slimmers make is to think that eating in order to be a healthy weight is in some way a punishment. The day we stop thinking that way is the day that long-lasting and painless weight loss can begin.

6
Weight Loss That Works

This chapter is a straightforward set of suggestions, based on a combination of my own experience of what works and what doesn't in the long term and international research studies and scientific evidence. It doesn't involve weighing and measuring of foods, fiddling about, lots of extra time or effort, separate meals, strange eating patterns or guilt-inducing strategies. It is all about portion control, coupled with weight-control friendly foods in the right balance and at regular intervals.

The Truth About Calories

Calorie counting as a means to losing weight went out of favour back in the last century sometime (circa 1990, if I remember). But while it is true that actual 'calorie counting' is not an ideal way to reduce calorie intake, the fact is that calories *do* count.

A two-year study funded by the National Institutes of Health recruited hundreds of overweight people and assigned each of them to one of four diets, each with a different macronutrient profile (from low-fat to high-fat and from moderately low-carb to high-carb; all the diets were low in saturates and high in fresh produce and fibre). The participants were supposed to eat no fewer than 1200 calories a day and take regular exercise. In six months, the dieters lost around 6kg (13lb), no matter which diet they followed. So as long as a diet reduces calorie intake enough to create an energy deficit, it will result in weight loss.

However, while calories do count, they may not be the only factor in losing weight or staying slim, as we've seen and will see some more. So let's ignore (at least for most of the time) the kitchen scales and the detailed calorie books, and forge a compromise ...

The 40:30:30 balance

We've already seen that the official advice is that you should eat about 50 per cent of your diet as carbohydrates. In fact, both in the UK and USA we eat nearer 55 per cent.

If you are trying to lose weight, my suggestion is that you take that level down to around 40 per cent. Crucially, you should achieve most of this by reducing your sugar and high-GI foods intake.

New research funded by the US Institutes of Health backs up the reduced-carb philosophy. A diet of 43 per cent carbs reduced insulin, stabilised blood sugars and creating a full feeling for longer after a meal. And, 'Over the long run, a sustained modest reduction in carbohydrate intake may help to reduce energy consumption and facilitate weight loss,' one of the study authors said.

The reduction in carbohydrate intake will allow you to eat more protein (about 30 per cent of your total calories), which, we have seen, is something of a star in the weight-control field, as it improves satiety and speeds up the metabolic rate. It also allows you to eat plenty of the 'healthy' fats – 30 per cent again.

Furthermore, a 2008 review published in the journal *Current Opinion in Endocrinology, Diabetes, and Obesity* concluded that 'diets moderately increased in protein and modestly restricted in carbohydrate and fat, particularly saturated fat, may have beneficial effects on body weight, body composition, and associated metabolic parameters'.

I believe from all that I have witnessed over the past years, a 40:30:30 balance of the major nutrients is ideal for slimming. (You will notice I haven't mentioned alcohol, the macronutrient we don't need, but which most of us do take – more on that to come.)

FORTY PER CENT CARBS – THE GUIDELINES
- The majority of the carbs you eat should be low or medium–low GI.
- Your carbs should be healthy and whole.
- Avoid refined 'white' carbohydrates.
- Keep your sugar intake low – no more than 20 per cent of your total carbs, and nearer 10 per cent would be ideal. So on a slimming diet of around 1400 calories a day, that's equivalent to around 3–6 teaspoons of sugar.

It's important to understand that simply shifting the balance of your macronutrients slightly will not result in weight loss, unless that shift produces a reduction in your energy (i.e. calorie) consumption. However, I believe that eating the right balance of the right types of food will, naturally and without bother, do exactly that for most people, most of the time, and will therefore result in the energy deficit required for weight loss. But if you are to achieve this, you'll need to get back in tune with your body's own signals and get your brain into gear (see Chapter Ten). Otherwise, you may follow the 40:30:30 principle, along with all the other advice in this chapter, and still not reduce your calorie intake by even 1 per cent.

✱ *An example*
In actual terms, let's see what a 40-30-30 plan looks like, on a day's typical slimming diet for a female.

TOTAL DAILY CALORIE INTAKE: **1400 CALORIES**
Of which:
40 per cent carbs 560 calories
(1g carbohydrate = 4 calories, so 140g per day carbs, comprising 30g –
maximum – sugars and 110g starches)
30 per cent protein 420 calories
(1g protein = 4 calories, so 105g protein per day)
30 per cent fat 420 calories
(1g fat = 9 calories, so 47g fat per day, comprising mainly polyunsaturated
and monounsaturated fats)

But do bear in mind that you don't need to weigh, measure, count grams or calories – this is just an example for your interest. Your own food intake may be more or less than the example above, depending on your size, activity levels, sex, age and so on. In general, the heavier you are, the more calories you can eat and still lose weight. As you lose weight, however, you may need to reduce your food intake pro-rata in order to continue losing weight. Regardless of your actual calorie intake, however, you should aim to keep the 40:30:30 balance.

Weight Control IQ – the Rules

1. Make the right choices of foods within each macronutrient group. In general, you are looking at low-GI, high-fibre carbs (including cereals, roots and pulses); lean proteins (from meat, dairy, fish,

eggs and soya); some fatty proteins (from oily fish, nuts and seeds and their oils); and a variety of different coloured vegetables, plus some low-GI fruits.

2. Eat three meals a day and two small snacks in between, spaced out fairly evenly. It may also help if your meals are all a similar size, as there is a fair amount of research to show that a good breakfast helps prevent snacking later in the day (but as someone who rarely eats breakfast, I have to say that this theory doesn't work for everyone!).

3. At each lunch or supper meal, divide the plate into two halves. The first half should contain a little over half carbohydrate food (e.g. potato) and the rest of it (a little under half) should contain lean protein food (or oily fish). The fat content of the meal will usually be hidden (oil in a dressing, for example, or butter on a potato, fat in cheese or meat and so on). The other half of the plate should be filled up with masses of vegetables or salad which, for the purposes of the 40-30-30 balance should be regarded as 'free' foods.

4. For meals which you can't separate – e.g. a stew or soup or pasta dish – simply use your commonsense, both in cooking and in serving, to follow the 40-30-30 guidelines.

5. At each breakfast meal, follow the same protein/carb rule (e.g. yogurt and muesli, Weetabix and skimmed milk) and finish the plate off with a good helping of fresh fruit (and some dried fruit if you like), plus a sprinkling of nuts and/or seeds for fat.

6. At each snack meal, choose a small, low-GI piece of fruit (see p. 86), plus a small piece of lean protein (natural yogurt, a square of cheese or a small slice of chicken, for example) or a few nuts or seeds.

7. Don't eat until you feel slightly hungry (not ravenous). If you find you are not hungry for three meals and two snacks a day, reduce your portion sizes (across the macro board) at each meal until you do, rather than skipping meals or snacks.

8. Eat slowly. According to Japanese studies carried out in 2008, fat people eat faster than slim people. Those who eat fast eat more because their 'feel full' mechanisms have not had time to kick in. So chew, then chew again and savour. Concentrate on the act of eating. Enjoy it. In fact, if you eat as I've recommended above, you will eat more slowly quite naturally – test and see how long it takes you to eat an apple (60 calories), compared with one small chocolate (80 calories).

9. Eat plenty of raw foods and 'large pieces', so that you have to chew – both will increase your DIT (see p. 70).

10. And, almost the most important of all: exercise portion control (see box below). Portion sizes have increased side by side with our growing obesity, and a 2009 US study showed that adults who tried portion control as a way to reduce weight lost 5 per cent more weight than people who tried other methods, such as low-fat diets.

A WORD ABOUT HUNGER

If you want to lose weight, then learn to enjoy feeling hungry. It's not as mad as it sounds. When you allow yourself to get hungry before you eat, you will appreciate healthy foods much more. An apple can be rather boring if you're full up, but if you're hungry, it tastes delicious. Don't be frightened of mild hunger pangs: once upon a time, they were normal. (For more on hunger and appetite, see Chapter Ten.)

PORTION CONTROL

- Always remember the protein/carb/vegetables (or fruit) ratio explained in rule 3 above, and never stint on size of portions for vegetables.
- Give yourself slightly less of a protein food that is higher in fat (Cheddar cheese, oily fish, lamb chops, for example) than the lean proteins (white fish, skinless chicken) and increase your vegetable serving to compensate.
- Think of the money you are saving by having two slices of roast beef instead of three, or a 25g piece of farmhouse Cheddar rather than a 50g piece.
- Put less on your plate than you think you will need. If, five minutes after you have finished what was on your plate, you are still genuinely hungry, take a little more.
- Portion control is much easier if you use smaller plates and dishes and if you only cook what you are intending to eat (or, for convenience, cook and freeze extra portions).
- Use smaller packages of food (research shows we take more from a larger pack of pasta, rice or cereal, for example, than we do from smaller ones. If this isn't practical (say, you have a large family), decant into smaller bags.

How will you know if you are getting your energy intake/output balance right?

OK, I hear you say, if I'm not counting calories or weighing food how do I know I am not still eating too much?

Well, that one is quite easy. Simply take your waist measurement once a week using a tape measure and see if it's going down. A centimetre (half an inch) a week, and you're doing fine. Also, see if your clothes feel a bit looser. Once in a while – if you must – weigh yourself and see if the weight is going down.

If, after 2–3 weeks, you find you have not lost or have stopped losing weight, your first port of call is to decrease your portion sizes a little more with a particular eye on the carbs (especially sugars). And keep remembering the hunger thing (see p. 98) – it's a really good indicator. You may also need to increase your activity levels (see Chapter Nine).

To continue making an energy deficit and to continue losing weight, you need fewer calories (and/or more activity). Make sure you eat enough protein – this will help keep your lean mass and metabolic rate up too.

Finally, take a look at the amount of fat you're eating. While you don't want to be on an actual low-fat plan, you need to remember to keep it within 30 per cent of your total calorie intake. Because fat is so high in calories, it's easy to lose track of your intake, so if the weight loss isn't happening or has slowed down, take slightly fewer nuts for your snack, pour a little less olive oil dressing on your salad, cut most of that fat band off your steak or chops, skim that

---

TOP TEN FOODS AND DRINKS FOR HELPING WEIGHT CONTROL THE HEALTHY WAY

1 Lean protein foods, to speed up metabolism and promote satiety.
2 Low-GI carbs, to stave off hunger and stabilise blood sugar.
3 Low-fat dairy, to increase fat metabolism and stabilise blood sugar.
4 Omega-3 fats, to reduce body fat and insulin resistance.
5 Calcium-rich foods, to reduce fat absorption and hunger.
6 White and green teas, to increase fat burning.
7 Watery foods, to cut overall calorie consumption.
8 Spices, such as chilli, to boost metabolic rate by up to 20 per cent and give important flavour sensation.
9 Herbs, again to add flavour without calories.
10 Crunchy and raw foods that need chewing, such as a fresh apple, a crisp salad or some nuts, to help satiety and (according to research) improve mood.

obvious fat off the top of your curry. Go back and read about good and bad fats again (see p. 88) and reduce the 'bad' ones first.

You might also need to review what you're drinking (see pp. 90–1).

SOYA BEANS TO LOSE WEIGHT?
Researchers in Seoul fed rats a high-fat, high-black-soya-bean diet and found they gained half as much weight as the rats fed a high-fat diet without the beans. The mechanisms of this fat-blocking effect are not well understood yet, though the metabolism-boosting effect of the protein in the beans may be a factor.

Shopping IQ

Most of us go to a food shop to buy certain things – and come out with several extra items we had no intention of buying at all. Good result for the shop – bad result for us and our waistlines.

Although more space in our major stores is now being devoted to fresh vegetables, salads and fruits, meat and fish, the best profit margins are still in the highly processed food aisles: the soft drinks, cans, packets, jars and so on. Unfortunately, that's usually where the most calories, fat and sugar are too.

An awareness and understanding of the ploys that supermarkets use to tempt you can help to prevent you from buying the things you – and your body – do not need. This section will equip you with shopping IQ; remember, IQ is knowledge, and the intelligence to use that knowledge.

Here are some of the most common retailing strategies:

- Super-large trolleys: the big space inside tempts you to buy more.
- Placing top brands in the middle of aisles: you have to walk past a lot of other stuff to reach the brand you want, so that something else catches your eye along the way and you stop and put it in the trolley.
- In smaller shops, essentials such as bread and milk, are placed right at the back of the shop, so again, you see more goods on the way that you are more likely to buy on impulse.
- Point-of-sale displays. Many stores place chocolate, sweets and crisps near the checkout, so you pick them up while you are waiting to pay.
- Reduced prices for bulk items. You wanted a four-pack of buns, but there are twelve for only double the price of four, so you buy them.

You've got a lot of buns you don't need and the supermarket has got more of your money.

- Two for the price of one. Sounds like a great bargain, but only if you actually need two.
- Coupling. You go to the salad counter to buy fresh lettuce, for example, and see a bottle of ready-made Caesar dressing and packets of croutons beside it. You had no intention of buying these, but you do.

And some shopping IQ tips to evade them:

- Write a list before you go shopping.
- Go shopping when you are not hungry. If you are hungry, you will definitely buy more.
- Concentrate on not getting distracted by items you weren't going to buy. Move around the shop as quickly as you can. According to a population study once you pick something up and look at it, there is a 50 per cent chance you will buy it.
- Only buy bulk and two-for-one offers if you know you can use the extra − for example, if you can freeze it, share it with a neighbour or if it has a long use-by date, so it will keep until it is legitimately needed.
- If possible, shop at stores where there is less choice. Less choice means less temptation, saving you money, calories and even time.

Special dieters' foods

One of the problems with special 'diet' foods is that manufacturers often remove fat, but keep in a lot of sugar, and there may also be long lists of rather unnatural-sounding ingredients, if you check the labels.

While there is a place for manufactured products with less total fat than before and with less sugar, salt and, perhaps, calories, these should be everyday products that everyone might buy, and not products marketed for slimmers. For more information about slimmers' foods, see pp. 67–8 and for manufactured food diets, see Chapter Seven.

What to ask yourself when shopping for food

- Will it make a positive contribution to a healthy diet (i.e. does it contain one or more 'good' points, such as high fibre, high vitamins, omega-3s)?

- Will it complement the items already in my larder/fridge?
- Is it reasonably natural – how much processing has it gone through? Or does the ingredients list include lots of E numbers and chemical-sounding names?
- Does the balance of calories, fat, protein and carbs on the nutrition label look good?
- Will I feel happy about purchasing it once I get home?
- Does my trolley/basket contain a good proportion of plant foods?

LOW-FAT SPREADS?

Did you know that reduced-fat spreads can still be up to 60 per cent fat, and that butter is only around 80 per cent fat, in any case?

In the UK the official classification is as follows:

Full fat	80–90 per cent fat
Reduced fat	41–60 per cent fat
Half fat	39–41 per cent fat
Low-fat/light	less than 39 per cent fat

As many manufactured margarine spreads have quite a long list of other ingredients, you may be just as well off choosing butter, but spreading it thinly (if the butter is at room temperature, not cold, this will make thin spreading much easier).

Cooking IQ

A notorious 2009 survey of the most popular cookbooks found that a high proportion of home-cooking recipes (and the top chefs are as guilty as anyone) are sky-high in fat and calories.

When you're following a recipe, don't follow blindly. If it seems to suggest too much fat, sugar or salt, for example, cut it down or use a substitute. So instead of double cream, for example, use low-fat crème fraîche or Greek yogurt. Unless you're baking (which is a bit of a science and if you don't get the proportions right it can fail), it won't be a disaster – you can always add more, but you can't take away.

Eating-out IQ

Most of us eat out occasionally in the evenings and possibly quite regularly, if you include takeaway lunches and snacks. Choices made in the café, sandwich bar, restaurant and pub can make a huge difference to how easy or hard it is to manage your weight and health through diet. So the more you eat out, the more important it is to make good choices from the foods on offer.

Here is my short ten-step guide to eating out, enjoying it and not feeling guilty afterwards:

1. Study the menu of your chosen restaurant before you book or go in. Most restaurants and chain takeaways have an online menu; some even include nutritional values. It is better to pick a place with healthy choices on the menu before you go, rather than arrive somewhere and find everything is a high-fat feast. (For high-end eating out you will usually find today that meals tend towards light and healthy, anyway, so this is less of a problem.)

2. Consider cuisine type. Those which tend towards the healthy end of the spectrum include Japanese and vegetarian Indian. Modern British/French with its smaller portions are useful and have the potential to be healthy, but my main moan here is that you don't get enough vegetables/fibre. Most other types may have healthy selections, but also non-healthy.

    You may feel that a vegetarian or wholefood/organic restaurant or lunch stop may be perfect, but in my own experience, meals at the wooden-table cafés can be just as high in saturated fats, salt, calories etc. as in the local fast-food outlet. The quality of produce may be more to your liking, and there may be more vegetables/ pulses in the meal, but if you're watching your waistline, there may be little that is better for you beyond the fact that they may have a lower glycaemic index.

3. Make considered choices. Wherever you are eating, there is nearly always a selection of better dishes to go for, in terms of lower in calories/total fat, sugars, salt etc. There are moves to make restaurants display this information on their menus but until that happens mostly you can only make informed guesses, but that is better than nothing.

4. Don't think that places that offer 'starters only', tapas or similar are going to be better. Remember the buffet mentality (see p. 37) – the

more variety of food on offer, the more you are likely to eat. For a similar reason, avoid the self-serve 'all you can eat' salad buffets and carveries unless a) you aren't hungry and/or b) you have gone through all the psychological pointers in this book and come out the other side.

5. At a traditional restaurant, think about having one course only. Starters are easy to dispense with; or order two starters instead of a starter and a main meal. If you have chosen a place with a mouth-watering selection of desserts, try sharing with your partner, and convince yourself it is the taste experience you are there for, not the amount.

6. Fast food and takeaways: some fast-food chains have made efforts to improve their nutritional profile, so you should be able to find at least one or two items on most menus that are OK (and I'm only talking about nutritional profile here – you'll have to make up your own mind about quality, environmental issues and so on; or read my *Green Food Bible* to help you decide). If you only eat in these places once in a while it doesn't really matter what you choose (but picking the smaller sizes is still a good idea), but if it is a regular event, it is very easy to put on weight if you aren't careful. For regular users I suggest checking out the nutritional details of the meals and sides and drinks online – you may get quite a shock. Although some still don't disclose these details, which I find tells its own story. Independents are a worse minefield – think of the local chippie, pie shop, Indian takeaway … you'll never know how many calories and how much fat is in the fare on offer, but believe me, it will be a lot.

7. Sandwich bars and supermarket takeouts. Beware: just because it's a sandwich or it's cold, doesn't mean it isn't a potential waist-expander. Similarly, because it's a salad, doesn't mean it's healthy or low in calories. Mayonnaise is a high-fat, high-calorie food, so why choose egg mayo with crisp leaves and shredded carrot salad? The bare truth is that popping into a retail outlet for your snacks or meals is a minefield, and if you value knowing exactly what you're eating, it would be prudent to get up ten minutes earlier and prepare a lunch to take with you. I do know that's not always practical though, so as a simple rule of thumb, check the label or check online before you buy. Again, if it's occasional, it may not matter what you choose. However, once you get into the healthy

eating mindset, it's preferable to pick the things that seem to offer the most nutrition for your money (see p. 82, for guidelines on what your body really needs).

8. If you buy lunch out, you should consider what you have/will be eating the rest of the day as well as your personal circumstances. Take a 1.8m (6ft) tall male who rushes around all day, for example: if he has fruit and low-fat yogurt for breakfast and will have a piece of steamed salmon, plus a huge quantity of stir-fried mixed vegetables (fried in a tad of groundnut oil) for supper, he might be better off going for the calorie-laden baguette rather than the dainty crayfish and yogurt salad (no mayo) with melon to follow for lunch. (Not least because the crayfish and melon choice will surely be followed, before long, by a large Mars bar due to hunger pangs.)

9. Think about drink. Sipping water in between wine is a good way to reduce your alcohol intake.

10. Whenever you're eating anywhere other than your own home, remember the weight control IQ rules on pp. 96–8. Eat slowly, savour each mouthful etc. It really does help.

AN AT-A-GLANCE GUIDE TO EATING OUT

Cuisine	Go for
Italian	Liver, veal, vegetables, shellfish, sardines, starter portions of pasta with vegetable sauces
French	Provençal vegetable dishes, seafood, sorbets
Indian	Tandoori bakes and grills, dhals and lentil curry, basmati rice
Thai	Chilli crab or prawns, hot and sour dishes
Spanish	Tortilla, salads, fish, soups
Chinese	Chicken, prawn, tofu stir-fries
Japanese	Most sushi is a good choice
Greek/Turkish	Lean meat kebabs with vegetables or salad
Moroccan/North African	Lamb/apricot or chicken/lemon tagines, salads, bulgur

Note: research shows that eating a lot of monosodium glutamate – frequently added to many Chinese takeaway meals – can hinder weight loss and encourage fat gain, a potential reason being that it may suppress fat breakdown in the body.

FACT

You may be interested to know that wherever you go to eat (and that includes buying a sandwich, ready meal or salad from the supermarket) that calorie counts are only an estimate – research has shown that the figures given are out by up to 20 per cent.

We all (and that definitely includes me) love to eat out, if we can afford it, sometimes, so the idea here is not to reduce the experience to a miserable, pointless exercise, but to help you wake up the next morning thinking what a wonderful meal and evening you had, rather than feeling guilty and bloated.

In conclusion, true body IQ includes the acceptance that the modern high-sugar, high-fat, high-salt, highly processed diet will probably not keep you slim, unless you happen to be a male teenager and/or someone who is physically extremely active most of your waking hours. And even if it does keep you slim, such a diet is unlikely to keep you healthy in the long term. You need to eat good, healthy food, as described above, and you need to learn to love it to succeed.

You also need to acknowledge that many of the diets you will find in packets, on the internet, in private clinics, in books and elsewhere are unlikely to be the saviours you seek – most certainly not in the long term. That is why I devote the next chapters to dissecting diets and slimming treatments that aim to part you from your cash.

When that is done, your body IQ should be strong, complete and ready – ready for the escape from the fat trap for good.

7
Diets Dissected

We've talked a lot about food – what's good, what's less good, what makes a 'balanced' diet and what will help you have a healthy body and maintain a good weight.

We've also touched on the thorny problem of fad diets, quick-fix dieting and how they don't help you escape from the fat trap – or, indeed, from the tyranny of skinny. Part of the problem is that there are just so many different methods to choose from, each claiming their way is 'the best'. Even I, who have been studying diets, dieting and the diet industry for years, get confused; so it's no wonder the ordinary person who just wants to lose a bit of weight and feel better feels mystified and is often hoodwinked by all the headlines and claims.

In this chapter, we're going to look at a few of the most popular diets on the planet and see just why – or if – they are so bad.

But first …

… What is a Diet?

Diet, in general terms, means 'what you eat'. Indeed, I am often known as 'the diet detective' because I enjoy analysing what and why we eat. But in the past few decades, the word 'diet' has come to be known as something you do when you want to lose weight. And 'dieting' never sounds like fun – it always sounds like a penance, a chore, a burden, even a withdrawal.

So many reasons why our hearts and spirits sink around the D-word. Yet, we continue to do it – time and time again – and the diet industry in all its guises continues to thrive as a result.

Approach With Caution!

You don't need 'a diet' in order to reach or maintain a good body weight. You just need to adjust your food intake and your activity output, as we've seen.

The on-/off-a-diet mentality is the exact opposite of good body IQ and is what prevents you from escaping the fat trap. It's why 95 per cent of people who 'diet' are back to their previous weight (and have mostly gained more) within a few years. And it's why I have reached the conclusion that almost any short-term 'diet plan', even if it is based on good, healthy food and healthy-eating principles, should be approached with caution.

As with all rules, of course, there may be exceptions. There are times when a couple of days eating not much and drinking plenty of water may make you feel better about yourself (say, after a week's eating and drinking a bit too much over Christmas or on holiday) and able to start on more measured habits again. Or sometimes, medics will require clinically obese people to lose a lot of weight quite rapidly to prepare them for, say, an operation. In this case, the strict diet and rapid weight loss are justified because they are less risky than staying obese and not having the op.

But for most of us, there is no pressing need to shed a certain amount of weight in a certain time, and nothing clever about doing so when we know that nine out of ten times we will put it back on.

All that being said, let's now look at some of those famous and popular 'diets' and see how well or how poorly they fit in with body IQ, and what they may do for you. At the end of each section I give the diet in question a 'Dieting Intelligence Quotient' (DIQ) rating based on their health, safety, effectiveness, palatability, sense and user-friendliness (rated on a scale of 1–5 stars).

So, is *any* of them worth trying? Let's see.

ARE YOU A SERIAL DIETER?

If you are a serial dieter, sit down at a computer or grab a piece of paper and, if you can, work out how many times you have lost weight. Then, think of a rough average amount of weight you've lost each time and work out the total you've lost over the years. Now, do the same with the amount you put back on. You will probably come up with a figure of many kilograms of weight lost and regained. And for what?

The moral: lose weight slowly, by eating along the lines suggested in Chapter Six and, if you are tempted by a 'diet', remember … the more weight loss promised and the shorter the time span, the wider berth you should give it (unless your doctor tells you differently, in which case you should be supervised to lose weight, anyway).

High-protein Diets

These first caused a stir in the USA and UK in the 1970s, disappeared, then came back in a huge way in the '90s when Dr Atkins, one of the major pioneers of high-protein-eating to lose weight, revived his Diet Revolution and turned it into big business. There have been several other high-protein diets and books along the way.

Dr Atkins New Diet Revolution, Dr Robert C. Atkins (Vermilion, 2003)

✱ *What it is*

A very high-protein, high-fat, very low-carbohydrate diet which was updated from the original *Diet Revolution* book of the 1970s back in 2003.

A typical day's diet on the two-week 'induction' phase would be fried egg and bacon for breakfast, coffee with cream; chicken and salad greens with olive oil dressing for lunch; steak and salad greens with mayonnaise for supper with a between-meal snack of ham slices.

On average the diet contains around 1200–1500 calories a day, comprising 75g fat, 35g saturates, 125g protein, under 20g carbs and 2–5g fibre.

✱ *The claims*

The premise is that the diet works to produce rapid weight loss (1.8–5.4kg/ 4–12lb in fourteen days), not because it is low in calories – you can 'eat all you like' of the allowed foods – but because the lack of carbs and the huge amount of protein create a natural state of fat-burning in the body, speeding up the metabolic rate and dampening hunger by causing ketosis (see p. 110). It also claims that avoiding carbs decreases insulin production and this means that insulin resistance (see p. 69) is avoided.

✱ *The facts*

As we've seen in Chapter Six, a diet moderately high in protein can be a help for people who want to lose weight as it can increase the metabolic rate and helps prevent hunger. But the *New Diet Revolution* goes to extremes. A typical choice of menu provides virtually no carbs, at least three times as much protein as is needed for adults and a lot more fat than guidelines recommend, at about 50 per cent or more (half of which is saturates).

And not all studies show that the *very* low-carb, high-protein plan promotes greater or faster weight loss, either. In one study (*American Journal of Clinical*

Nutrition), obese participants followed either a very low-carb (5 per cent) diet equivalent to Atkins' 20g a day or a 40 per cent carb diet. After six weeks, the two groups had lost similar amounts of body fat and weight. The very low-carb diet was also linked with several adverse metabolic changes. As a result, the researchers recommend avoiding very low-carb diets. This is only one small study, but several facts do seem clear:

- The diet does produce ketosis. This is the process used to convert body fat into energy. If you consume fewer calories than your body requires, first you'll use up glycogen stored in your liver, then you'll start to use body fat. When this fat is broken down, the resulting fatty acids are used by your liver to produce ketones. These are a water-soluble form of energy that can be used by most tissues as fuel. Ketones can also pass across the blood–brain barrier to be used by your brain. Being in ketosis can indeed reduce appetite and people often feel more alert and energetic. However, it usually gives bad breath and can cause other problems (see below).
- The Atkins diet almost certainly will produce a daily reduction of calorie intake which is the real main reason for any weight loss. Although high-cal foods such as butter, cream and mayo are not, in theory, limited, because items such as potatoes, pasta and bread are banned, opportunities to eat these high-cal foods are automatically drastically reduced. (e.g. no more cheese sandwiches or eggs on toast).
- The other way the diet reduces calories is by inducing boredom. As tempting as unlimited meat can sound (especially to men), it does become dull before too long – there is only so much steak or eggs you can eat without chips or a baked potato.
- A high-protein, low-carb diet encourages the body to excrete fluid, and so there will be several kilograms lost in water during the early stages of the diet.

✱ *Health and safety*

The diet is very low in fibre which is important for digestive health and disease prevention; a high saturated-fat diet is still linked with increased risk of cardiovascular disease and the strict banning of most of the fruits and many of the vegetables and grains that we are actually encouraged by health officials to consume more of, is maverick. The antioxidants and other chemicals found in plant foods are vital for disease prevention, so limiting their intake – along with the range of vitamins and minerals found in fruits, grains and vegetables – is risky.

A diet very high in meat may leach calcium from the bones and increase the risk of osteoporosis. It also raises environmental issues.

The state of ketosis (see above) can be dangerous. It can cause irritability, headaches, stress on the kidneys, palpitations and even a heart attack.

✱ Conclusion

While many people did – and undoubtedly still do – lose weight easily and successfully following the Atkins diet and similar regimes, it is hard to come out in favour of any plan that is extreme and which flies in the face of current nutritional and medical thinking on the amounts of saturated fat and plant foods that we should consume.

Indeed, the diet would be very hard for vegetarians to follow, and impossible for vegans. Talking of which, if a very high-protein, high-fat, very low-carb regime is the right way to lose weight and stay slim, why, according to several population studies, are vegans the slimmest group of people on the planet?

This eating regime is, in effect, a fad diet, and as the science behind it is flawed in places, it would make more sense to follow a more moderate diet (along the lines recommended in this book, or one of those described on pp. 135–8), and not run the risk of nutritional imbalances.

DIQ: ★★

✱ *The New High Protein Diet* by Dr Charles Clark and Maureen Clark, revised edition (Vermilion, 2007).
Similar type of diet with a similar rationale, but allowing up to 60g (2½oz) carbs in the weight-loss phase and with a better selection of recipes.
DIQ: ★★★⌐

✱ *Curves: Permanent Results Without Permanent Dieting* by Gary Heavin and Carol Colman (Century, 2003).
Similar to Atkins, but lower in fat, with 20g (¾oz) carb max or 60g (2½oz) carb max options.
DIQ: ★★★

Detox Diets

Detox diets appear to be thriving, despite the plethora of material indicating that they don't help detoxify the body or produce long-term weight loss and may be harmful to health. Many are endorsed – or at least used – by celebrities, such as Victoria Beckham, Gwyneth Paltrow and Beyoncé, and that could be one reason for their popularity.

Since I last looked at the detox market, there are several 'new' ones, albeit mostly based on the old, worn, unproven theories. Here are some of the most popular – starting with a close look at the famous lemon detox.

The Lemon Detox Diet

✱ *What it is*

This detox diet – sometimes called the Maple Syrup Diet or the Neera Supercleanse – is one of the world's top-selling detox regimes, with half a million litres of the syrup sold a year, and is said to have helped singer Beyoncé lose 10kg (22lb) in fourteen days.

You buy a 1-litre (1¾-pint) tin of 'tree syrup', the contents of which is a mix of palm and maple syrups, to which you add fresh lemons, cayenne and water and drink 1800ml (3 pints) or six glasses a day. You can buy just the can, or complete kits.

The £79.90 kit from www.slimmingsolutions.co.uk contains the syrup, a bottle of cayenne, a piece of ginger and seven lemons, as well as, for some reason, fifty 'slimming tea' bags. Following the make-up instructions, the syrup would last seven days and the lemons just over two days. There are various books, of which Dr K. A. Beyer's *The Lemon Detox Diet: Rejuvenation Sensation* (PNP, 2006) is one of the most popular and often sold with kits. He also recommends buying bee pollen to take for two months.

✱ *The claims*

You will lose 3–5.4kg (7–12lb) in ten days without feeling hungry. Also claims many health benefits, including elimination of allergies, colds, flu, sinusitis, bronchitis, joint problems, skin infections and an increase in the 'elasticity of the body'.

✱ *The facts*

A few quotes from Beyer's book and the kit blurb:

'The majority of illnesses originate in the digestive system which is often overloaded. Food is not well digested and waste products and toxins accumulate.'

Um, no – the majority of illnesses don't originate in the digestive system, and the digestive system copes well with digesting food, that's what it is for. The body defends itself well against most toxins – from the environment and overeating, for example, additive- or pesticide-rich foods – and, in any case, as toxins are stored in body fat, a short-term diet isn't going to eliminate them all. It's long-term healthy habits and maybe changes in lifestyle (even in where you live perhaps) that will do this. Waste products are eliminated in the normal way and, as we see below, this diet can actually cause constipation which – if anything – would hinder, not help elimination.

'White sugar is almost completely lacking in energy – the body needs nutrients (such as B vitamins and calcium) to absorb it. White sugar causes damage to the teeth.'

In fact, sugar is easily digested by the body and converted to energy or fat, which is why it contributes to obesity. White sugar may cause damage to the teeth – but so does syrup of any kind, especially, as happens with this diet, if it is sipped as a sweet clingy drink during the day.

'No preservatives are added and no chemical processes are applied [to the syrup].'

However, the natural syrup from the palm trees would ferment if shipped as it is, so in fact, it is heated to drive off the moisture content, in effect turning it into palm sugar, which is then later turned back into syrup again with the addition of water.

'Waste products are deposited in the outermost cells of the body ...'

Wrong! Most of our waste products are processed and eliminated within the digestive system.

'... which includes those in the hair. For healthy hair, detoxification is absolutely necessary.'

Wrong again – on many levels. A short-term fast/diet of syrup and lemon is going to do nothing whatsoever for the health of hair.

'The fat just dissolves ... only this way can the great loss of weight be explained.'

Um – no. Body fat doesn't just dissolve into thin air when you drink syrup and lemon juice. It is converted in the usual way into usable energy to fuel the body which is not receiving much in the way of calories via your mouth. The 'great loss of weight' is explained by the fact that you are virtually fasting. For someone who is, say, 12.7kg (2 stone) overweight and has been eating around 2500 calories a day this extreme diet would give a daily deficit of around 2000 plus calories, which could result in a fat loss over ten days of nearly 2.7kg (6lb). Much of the rest will be water and some will be lean tissue.

'The vitamin C (in the lemon) is important as it acts as a preventative to rickets.' Rickets is a disease of the bones caused by vitamin D deficiency and no medical journal links it with a lack of vitamin C. Seems like Dr Beyer is confusing rickets and scurvy.

'The ascorbic acid (vitamin C) assists the cleansing process, acting as an internal detergent.' I can't find any scientific reference to vitamin C acting as an internal detergent.

So is there any truth in the claims? Well, it is almost sure to result in rapid short-term weight loss, as any very low-calorie diet will. The diet provides approximately 350 calories a day altogether – 313 in the syrup and 22 in the three lemons (equivalent to about 6 tablespoons of lemon juice). The syrup also provides around 72g (2½oz or 14 teaspoons) sugar, about an eighth of your day's calcium needs (yet they boast about its high calcium content), half of your zinc and some iron, magnesium and other minerals. The lemon provides around two thirds of the EC and USA RDA for vitamin C, and all of the UK's.

I won't try this diet myself, but I believe most people would feel hunger as, unlike a high-protein, low-carb diet, the lemon detox with its sugar content doesn't create a state of ketosis (see p. 110).

On the plus side, lemon juice has been shown to slow down the rate at which simple carbohydrates are absorbed into the bloodstream, so can help allay hunger pangs (but this effect would not be strong enough to counteract the hunger caused by the minimal calorie level). Palm sugar has a lower GI than common table sugar. And any low-calorie regime with no alcohol or starches can make you feel more alert and sharp. (But, of course, you could simply give up those things without doing the lemon detox.)

✱ Health and safety

For most people, 3–5.4kg (7–12lb) is an extreme amount to lose in ten days and could be unsafe, especially for ill or very active people or those with, for example, diabetes. Numerous studies have shown that fasting and extremely low-calorie intake – common features of most detox diets – cause a slowdown of metabolism and an increase in weight after the dieter returns to normal eating.

The book admits to constipation as a common side effect and suggests 2 teaspoons of salt in water a day to counteract this: that equals around 10g (½oz) salt, which is higher than the recommended daily maximum for adults according to the UK's Department of Health and the USDA. The alternative, as recommended in the book, is to take a daily laxative; however, these can cause more bowel problems than they solve.

This is a severe crash diet, likely to leave you not only hungry, but also lacking in energy, playing havoc with your blood-sugar levels. If you follow this diet for any length of time, you could end up with low nutrient levels, including iron, calcium, zinc and vitamin C. Lastly, a sugar/lemon juice combination can erode teeth and cause decay. (See also 'Drinks – why they could be keeping you fat', p. 90.)

✱ Conclusion

Much of the 'science' in both the book and the kit blurbs for the lemon detox is way out of line with what we know, and appears to be aimed at the gullible looking for a quick fix.

What you get is a high-sucrose drink with a bit of vitamin C and a few other nutrients, with no special magic except its low calorie content – all of which you could make yourself at home for a fraction of the cost.

At the end of the book, Dr Beyer lists several maxims by which you should live, including: Be sensible. Be practical. Be wise. Be careful. If you do, indeed, follow these four maxims, you probably won't want to buy into the lemon detox diet.

DIQ: ★

Clean: The Revolutionary Program to Restore the Body's Natural Ability to Heal Itself, Alejandro Junger MD (HarperOne, 2009; www.cleanprogram.com)

✱ What it is

A book containing details of a holistic 'detox' with much explanation as to why our lives and bodies need detoxing and why our systems need help to do this.

✱ The claims

Dr Junger says that a whole range of ills, including colds, viruses, allergies, obesity, insomnia, indigestion, skin conditions, depression and anxiety are all the 'direct result of toxic build-up in our systems accumulated through the course of our daily lives'. The programme can be easily incorporated into a busy schedule and the effect is transformative: nagging health problems will suddenly disappear, extra weight will drop away and, for the first time in our lives, we will 'feel healthy'.

His cleanse avoids 'acidifying foods', such as meat, dairy and sugar and one of his big enemies is mucus, which apparently covers all our cells if they get irritated by our toxic lifestyles. Like most promoters of detox diets, he says we are exposed to so many toxins that our bodies can't cope with them without help – a theory that is poo-pooed (forgive the pun!) by many health professionals.

✳ *The facts*

Clean is a complicated read and not for the faint-hearted. Dr Junger is a medical doctor and also an advocate of Eastern medicine, and his theories are often rooted in this. *Clean* is, in effect, an amalgamation of a digestive system detox, an allergy/elimination diet, a 'mind detox' (including meditation), lifestyle advice (including skin brushing, colonic irrigation and hot/cold plunge) and environmental advice (including installing an air-filtration system in the home and water filtration in the kitchen). Quite a daunting set of demands.

The clean-food programme gives you a liquid meal for breakfast, solid food at lunch time, another liquid meal for dinner, plus supplements. There is a high percentage of raw food, no dairy or eggs and only certain grains, though meat and fish are allowed. If you don't go to the loo every day you have to take laxative or caster oil. It also suggests a regular sandwich consisting of raw garlic between slices of apple.

✳ *Health and safety*

The permitted foods do provide a good range of nutrients and the recipes for smoothies, soups, juices and solid meals are varied (within the parameters of the rules). I estimate energy intake will be around 1000 calories a day and the plan lasts for three weeks. This is borderline–low, but there are no calories wasted on poor nutrient-quality foods, i.e. every calorie counts.

✳ *Conclusion*

A high-plant wholefood diet would probably benefit many of us and should be a good way to cut calorie intake easily. But I fear for most people living ordinary lives, the plan may be very hard to fit in to everyday existence, even for three weeks. If I were doing it, I would pick out the recipes and much of the food advice and quietly forget the rest – and still lose weight. I am also worried that the somewhat doom-laden messages in large parts of the book, about our toxic environment and food, may actually cause depression in some readers, rather than alleviate it. I am also quite irritated that after all the preaching in the book, the website appears to be a money-making tool, with the 'Clean Ultimate Kit' selling for $350 plus shipping costs. Complete with its plastic packaging. Isn't that toxic?

DIQ: ★★

7lbs in 7 days Superjuice Diet, Jason Vale (Harper Thorsons, 2006)

✱ What it is
Eat nothing, but drink juices for seven days and take additional supplements. The book contains recipes for the juices and motivational speak plus name-dropping from the author about how he helped the model Jordan to lose weight. Supplements recommended include spirulina and probiotics.

✱ The claims
Vale promises glowing skin, harder nails, increased pure raw energy levels (whatever they are), less stress and a whole list of other benefits, as well as the 3.2kg (7lb) weight loss in a week.

✱ The facts
Britons now consume over 2.2 billion litres of juice and juice drinks a year – around 36 litres (63 pints) for every man, woman and child. Juice is perceived as a healthy drink and, indeed, it can have some health benefits. For example, the fruits and vegetables used to make juices can reduce blood cholesterol, slow down prostate cancer, help prevent heart disease and Alzheimer's. But most types are higher in calories and sugar than people often realise.

As for nails – they will not grow hard in a week; it would take months to have any noticeable effect.

✱ Health and safety
Fruit juices only count towards one portion of your fruit and vegetables a day, no matter how much you drink, so the diet is four portions a day short on that count – surprising for a diet that includes nothing but fruit and vegetables!

A high-fruit-juice diet, especially if sipped over long periods, can contribute to tooth enamel erosion and decay.

A diet of juice only, unless based mostly on vegetable juices, which contain less sugar, may cause energy levels to fluctuate. (See p. 60 and p. 90 for more on why a high-juice diet may not be a particularly good idea.)

The superjuice diet is remarkably similar in nutritional composition to the Lemon Detox described above, if slightly better as vegetables are juiced too. Fruit juices are very high in sugars, as are palm and maple syrups, while lemons and most other fruit provide good levels of vitamin C. Juicing removes all fibre from the fruit, so it provides a quick rush of sugar to the blood – not an ideal way to diet.

If you want to diet on liquid fruit and vegetables, you would be much better off making smoothies – i.e. puréeing the whole fruit (peeled, as necessary). Then you get fibre, more antioxidants and other plant compounds, and you don't get the sugar rush.

✱ Conclusion

It's good that the diet completely avoids processed 'junk' food, but the benefits of juicing as opposed to eating the whole fruit or having a smoothie are nil. I'm worried that the drinks don't always taste good – a pity when the raw ingredients are often quite costly – because if a diet is even in part unpalatable, it is hard to stick to. Diets that have add-on supplements to buy are annoying too, plus you will need a good juicer for the recipes, which can be expensive (and a devil to clean). Lastly, you can't really eat out on the diet – Vale says take your flask of juice. As if your friends would appreciate that. In other words – clear the decks of your life, if you're doing this, it isn't a diet that sits well with a normal lifestyle at all.

DIQ: ★★

Sensible alternatives to detox diets

A week or two on a high organic-vegetable-and-fruit diet, with plenty of wholegrains, leafy greens, pulses, nuts and seeds; or try the Viva Mayr plan (see p. 127).

Meal-replacement Diets (MRDs)/ Very Low-calorie Diets (VLCDs)

Meal-replacement diets have been around since the 1980s, usually providing ready-made nutritionally counted shakes/bars/soups instead of a normal diet, or sometimes to be used for two meals a day with a normal calorie-counted meal in the evening (or other combinations depending on the company – most MRDs are franchises). MRDs that take the daily calories down lower than 800 a day and are the sole source of nutrition are called very low-calorie diets (VLCDs).

LighterLife

✱ What it is

A franchise. A combination of meal replacement diet/VLCD, plus weekly group counselling sessions, partly based on cognitive behavioural therapy (CBT). If you have 6.3kg (1 stone) or more to lose you can join. The cost, at the time of writing, is £66 a week. For people with a BMI over 25 there are three LighterLife (LL) food packs (which are all-liquid, either shakes or soups) and one 'conventional' meal, plus add-ons, such as a low-cal savoury broth or a fibre-rich, low-cal drink, bringing your daily calorie intake to 801 or more. For people with a BMI over 29 there are four LL food packs, containing 530 calories. 'Real' food is introduced gradually, towards the end of the programme.

* The claims

'Fast, simple, safe and sustainable, LighterLife is more than a diet. While you're losing weight, learn what's going on in your head so that you can keep the weight off.'

LighterLife say on their main website that their counsellors have to pass a BTEC professional certificate or diploma in weight-management consultancy, and that this qualification is of equal educational standard to a level 4 NVQ or a foundation degree.

* The facts

One hundred and fifty thousand people have done LighterLife. As with most meal replacement/VLCD programmes, the weight comes off quickly and most participants would agree that it is fast and simple (the safety angle is discussed in the general conclusions below).

Whether the weight loss is sustainable, however, is another matter. In June 2009, the Advertising Standards Authority adjudication on a TV advertisement for LighterLife, which had been the subject of viewer complaints, said: 'We considered that viewers were likely to interpret [the woman in the advertisement's] statement ... to mean that the VLCD was a long-term solution to obesity itself. Because it was not, we concluded the ad was misleading. We welcomed LighterLife's assurance that their ads would not refer to long-term solutions in future.'

However, the weekly counselling and the fact that LL encourage people who have slimmed on their programme to return to their management sessions regularly should be a plus point and very helpful.

* Health and safety

LighterLife offers diet support and counselling at a weekly group meeting, and the company's boasts about their counsellors' qualifications (see above) encourage a sense of security in the advice and support that will be provided. But in the franchise pack it says they can start up 'within four months' and then 'have the opportunity to be accredited by Edexcel with a BTEC Diploma in Weight Management Consultancy'. Having the opportunity is not the same as actually having the BTEC when they start up, surely? Elsewhere, they say all their counsellors are 'working towards' an accredited Edexcel diploma. As BTEC diplomas equivalent to a foundation degree normally take a year to complete with almost full-time study, it cannot be the case that all new recruits to LighterLife counselling (who are expected, as explained in the franchise brochure, to put in around thirty-five hours a week simply running the LL business) have this qualification at the outset.

LL are adamant that participants on the VLCD are required to get a health questionnaire completed and signed by a doctor, acknowledging that the patient is taking part in the programme. (Most doctors charge a fee for this service.) However, in the LighterLife franchise presentation document it clearly states ' ... counsellors will ask clients to complete a health questionnaire. Depending on their health, a client may need their questionnaire filled out by a GP.' LL also say clients must have a health check (which the client is responsible for organising and paying for as necessary) every twenty-eight days.

As I couldn't get any answers from LighterLife's headquarters, I put out a media request on the huge Netmums website asking for people who had been on the LL programme to contact me. I checked with those who did, and all had indeed been asked to get a doctor's signature, and most were happy with their experience of LL.

However, getting a doctor's OK before beginning is not the same thing as 'under medical supervision', which is how most health bodies describe VLCDs should be undertaken – the counsellors have no requirement to have any medical training.

In June 2009, after an adjudication by the Advertising Standards Authority cast doubt on the medical supervision aspects of the programme, LighterLife were told by the ASA 'not to target obese people unless the treatment was conducted under adequate medical supervision'. As VLCDs are – or should be – aimed at the clinically obese, I could say that LL seem to have a problem ...

Regarding nutritional quality, the VLCD programme contains 100 per cent of the recommended daily amounts of all the nutrients for which the Department of Health UK provides RDAs. However the DoH gives no RDAs for plant chemicals, including antioxidants, which are a major factor in protecting us from disease. To help prevent constipation, a frequent problem on a VLCD of any type, more water or other fluids than normal should be consumed – from 2–4 litres a day, spread out evenly.

And see my conclusions on VLCDs, below.

DIQ: ★★

The Cambridge Diet (www.cambridge-diet.co.uk)

Cambridge has been going since 1984 and has different levels of calorie intake from 415 a day up to 1500. It is sold only through 'counsellors' (in fact, franchisees) who you see in person, one to one, and who monitor progress. According to users, the weekly cost, at the time of writing, works out at about £40 (though, strangely, the franchises can charge what they want, so costs will vary).

One concern is that they say the 810-calories-a-day diet is suitable for 'anyone above BMI 20 who is not medically contraindicated'. Does anyone with a BMI of just 20 really need to be losing weight, let alone on 810 calories a day?

According to the Cambridge website, Sole Source® (415 calories) and Sole Source Plus® (615 calories) can be used for rapid weight loss only by people with 'a BMI of 25 plus a stone'. I emailed Cambridge to ask what this means and how one works it out and didn't receive a reply.

Here are the ingredients in a Cambridge Diet chocolate-flavour meal-replacement bar containing 172 calories; 57 per cent of its 5.8g fat content (including hydrogenated fat) is saturated.

Chocolate flavour: Maltitol syrup, Milk chocolate (Sugar, cocoa butter, dried whole milk, cocoa mass, whey powder, emulsifier: soya lecithin, flavouring), Whey protein concentrate, Whey powder, Milk protein, Fat reduced cocoa powder, Hydrogenated palm oil, Potassium chloride, Sodium pyrophosphate, Calcium carbonate, Soya lecithin, Calcium phosphate, Magnesium hydroxide, Emulsifier (E472b), Ascorbic acid, Ferrous fumarate, Copper gluconate, Nicotinamide, Zinc oxide, Vitamin E acetate, Manganese sulphate, Calcium D pantothenate, Pyridoxine hydrochloride, Thiamine hydrochloride, Riboflavin, Vitamin A acetate, Chromic chloride, Sodium molybdate, Folic acid, D biotin, Vitamin K, Potassium iodate, Sodium selinate, Vitamin D3, Vitamin B12.

I guess you either like to eat this kind of thing or you don't. I don't. But even if you do like it – it isn't re-educating your palate for decent, natural food, really, is it?
DIQ: ★★

Exante

Another franchise, this is a slightly less extreme diet than some, available mostly online or through a very few local 'consultants' and stockists. It comprises bars, shakes and soups, plus one meal a day, providing 1200

calories, or just three to four replacements a day to provide 600 or 800 calories. The website says you should not follow the 600/800-calorie-a-day diet unless your BMI is over 25, but as products are sold online, I am not sure how this can be monitored. The cost is £36.75 a week for twenty-one meal replacements.
DIQ: ★★

Weight to Go

Similar to Exante, but supplied with one 'proper' ready meal a day, which looks more like ordinary food and tastes OK. Plus, amazingly, you can add your own fresh fruit and vegetables! 850 calories a day; £55 for a week's supply.
DIQ: ★★↲

✱ *Conclusions on meal replacements/VLCDs*

Meal-replacement programmes have met with conflicting opinions from health bodies and the medical profession across the world. Some doctors see VLCD regimes as offering their obese patients an 'easy' way to slim (thus perhaps taking some of the pressure off them to offer more time-consuming ways to help, the cynic in me says).

Cambridge and Exante appear to allow users with a BMI of much less than 30 to use their VLCDs, which conflicts with the World Health Organisation advice which clearly states that VLCDs (fewer than 800 calories a day) should only be used for people with a BMI over 30, *under medical supervision.* Medical supervision doesn't happen in any accepted sense with these commercial VLCD franchises. Interestingly, the WHO also said that going below 800 calories does not, in any case, result in greater weight loss.

There have been deaths which have been linked to these programmes and reports (including unsolicited reports by participants on various internet chat rooms) of deteriorating eyesight, loss of periods in women, thinning hair, dizziness and various other problems, constipation being one of the most frequent side effects. Professor John Garrow, one of the UK's leading obesity specialists, has said: 'Studies show semi-starvation diets deplete the protein and muscle of internal organs, resulting in an increase of heart arrhythmias among obese people following them.' Although other scientific work shows that although lean tissue – including the heart – does shrink with significant weight loss, this doesn't harm heart function and may even improve it. As I explained back on p. 46, looking at individual studies does not always give the full picture.

Meal-replacement/very low-calorie diets usually produce rapid weight loss but, as with many diets, there is a high risk of weight regain, especially if no after-diet back-up or counselling is provided. But if counselling is provided, there need to be suitable checks in place to ensure the counsellor is properly trained and accredited before she or he begins the counselling sessions.

Food is supposed to be an enjoyable part of life. According to reviews these plans receive on the internet, many who have tried the 'meals' find them unenjoyable and unpalatable. Low-calorie meal replacements/VLCDs put proper food in a compartment labelled – 'do not touch at the moment'. I don't quite see how this fits in with LighterLife saying, for example: 'While you're losing weight, learn what's going on in your head so that you can keep the weight off.' It's one thing to think you know what's going on in your head when you don't actually have to deal with your food issues – another to put things into practice when they are once again a part of your daily life.

Meal replacements are another attempt to provide an easy option, a quick fix, a miracle cure for weight problems and obesity. They aren't about real food. *DIQ:* ★★

Sensible alternatives to meal replacements/VLCDs

If you are not constrained by cost, you could try one of the clutch of 'delivered diets' on offer in the UK; rather than synthetic meals, they provide you with proper 'real' food, delivered to your door, usually once a week. Of those I found, I prefer the meals at Pure Package (£32.95 a day for a 30-day programme, daily delivery); they sound delicious and well balanced, are ethical and include all your fresh vegetable and fruit requirements (whereas some others, such as Go Lower – £9.29 a day for 28-day plan – do not). Detox in a Box is OK (no red meat, wheat or dairy) at £16.50 a day, weekly delivery.

Or you could just try making your own simple, healthy meals in individual containers and freezing them. Use single-serve items such as sachets of porridge, pots of yogurt, pieces of fruit for breakfast and items such as ready-made 'healthy option' sandwiches or salads for lunch. Avoid alcohol, sugary drinks and snacking – voilà – a meal-replacement diet for a fraction of the cost!

Low-fat Diets

There are not many low-fat diets around any more; they fell out of favour in the late 1990s when Atkins made his major comeback and GI diets began their onslaught. However, some people still prefer this way of slimming and it is fairly flexible. The idea is that by reducing the fat content of your diet, you will lose weight without calorie counting, as fat, gram for gram, contains more calories than carbs or protein, and it is also the 'hidden' nutrient – slipping in your mouth and heading stomachwards almost without you noticing.

Both these facts are true, and as the recent USA research into different slimming diets found – a low-fat diet will help you to lose weight as long as you stick to it.

Slim to Win: Diet and Cookbook , **Rosemary Conley (Century, 2008)**

✱ *What it is*
Conley has produced some decent family-friendly recipes in the book and there's no bogus science – she marries low-fat with low-GI carbs to make the menus more satisfying and health-friendly.

✱ *Conclusion*
No major health or safety issues to worry about here. Still not enough good oils in here for my liking and protein content is a bit low compared with the conclusion I come to elsewhere in this book, but better than her early very low-fat books, and the very ordinariness of it all means it is more likely to have a good long-term outcome.
DIQ: ★★★★

Fad Diets

There is sometimes a thin line between what is a healthy diet, a fad diet and even a dangerous diet; the difference can be in the detail – the amount you're 'allowed' to eat, any strange supplements you are told to take and so on.

In preparing this list of what I have grouped as 'fads', I've included all kinds – from diets that have been around for thousands of years (and you may say, how can I call these fads?) – through those that target a particular body part and on to those that avoid whole food groups or are based on crazy 'science'. Other diets are just plain weird. The good news though is that they're not all bad.

Hay System (food combining)

I have to say that the Hay diet – possibly the original detox diet, invented over a hundred years ago by Dr William Hay and described in detail in several books in recent years – is much loved and practised by many people across the world.

✱ What it is
This is a diet that encourages you to avoid eating 'foods that fight' within your digestive system. Thus you should avoid eating carbs (which are broken down by alkaline saliva) and protein (needing gastric acid) at the same meal. You should also eat only whole foods, avoid refined starches, and follow a fairly long list of rules about how and how much you eat – e.g. fruit should always be eaten alone.

✱ The claims
Disease is caused by toxins and acid waste in the body and we can avoid this if we follow the Hay way of eating. No weight loss mentioned.

✱ The facts
The science behind the Hay idea is wrong. Not least because many healthy foods are a combination of both carbs and protein – pulses being an obvious example, wholegrains another. It would be impossible to avoid mixing carbs and protein in most normal meals. But people will lose weight on the system – if they are overweight and maybe even if they are not – as the rules will almost automatically reduce your food intake though not to extreme levels. As I have estimated, a day's average calorie intake, would be around 1000–1500.

✱ Health and safety
A wholefood diet avoiding refined starches is a great idea. Though it may be a little low on a few minerals, by and large it is a healthy and varied diet. No physical harm should come to followers by eating in the Hay way.

✱ Conclusion
Such a pity that a regime based on good, healthy eating is marred and muddied by a load of pseudoscience and overcomplicated rules, meaning that the diet won't be tried by many more people as it looks hard to fit into a normal life.
DIQ: ★★★

Blood Group Diet

A book by Dr Peter d'Adamo and Catherine Whitney (*Eat Right 4 Your Type* (Century, 1998)), proposing that you eat according to your blood group for health and weight loss; it was published just over ten years ago and the idea still sells.

✳ *What it is*

A range of diet plans based on the main idea that each of the four blood groups has its own unique 'antigen marker' and that this marker reacts badly with certain foods, leading to all sorts of potential health problems. Other complicated theories also come into play, but I won't bore you with those here.

✳ *The claims*

If you eat for your blood type, you will lose weight, have more energy, fight off infections, and protect yourself against disease and the ills of old age.

✳ *The facts*

There is no scientific research which concludes that your blood group has any bearing on how or what you should eat. It's also worth pointing out that the O, A, B method of classifying blood type is just one method of doing so – there are others. However, the diet will probably work to help most people lose weight, as for each of the groups, it is based on cutting out various foods and food groups which I estimate will result in an overall calorie intake reduction to around 1400–1500 a day.

✳ *Health and safety*

The main blood group type in the UK is O. The O-type diet is basically a high-protein, low-carb, dairy-free diet which could lead to nutrient deficiencies (for example, calcium). Type A is a relatively healthy plant and fish-based diet, type B is a high meat and dairy diet (not so great), while AB is a strange combination of A and B. Highly processed and refined foods are discouraged or banned, which is no bad thing, but the long list of decent, banned foods for each type means a balanced varied diet becomes more difficult to attain.

✳ *Conclusion*

No benefit for weight loss over other, easier, more straightforward diets. Could encourage faddy eating. The whole idea is based on a false premise.

DIQ: ★

The Cabbage Soup Diet

✱ What it is

Various forms of this pop up all over place, in books and on the internet. You basically make cabbage (and cabbage and vegetable) soup low in fat, protein and carbs, and eat it every day, plus one or two other 'allowed' foods (typically, fruit on day one, a baked potato on day two and so on).

✱ Conclusion

At around 800 calories a day, these diets are at (or close to) VLCD levels (see above), which are really only suitable for medically supervised obese people. But whereas at least with VLCDs the nutrient levels are regulated, on the cabbage diet you are likely to be low on protein and fat, B vitamins, calcium and other micronutrients, and it may also be high in salt, as the soups are often made with several stock cubes, which are one of the saltiest ingredients you can buy. Thus, despite getting most of their calories from vegetables (the only plus point, if there is one), these diets are not healthy at all.

DIQ: ★

The Viva Mayr Diet

✱ What it is

A fourteen-day diet and detox programme, designed by Dr Harald Stossier from the Viva Mayr clinic in Austria (where you can go to experience the regime for a few days for around £1000); it was also published as a book by Harper in 2009.

It is a strict regime involving 'intestinal cleansing' – no snacks; rather up to five hours between meals is recommended, as is 'breakfasting like a king' and having smaller lunches and suppers; chewing everything incredibly thoroughly, drinking bicarbonate of soda between meals, eating spelt bread and a list of healthy, whole foods including lots of organic vegetables, nuts, seeds, oils, fruits, spices, fish – and, surprisingly, some meat and dairy, though in small amounts.

✱ The claims

'Fourteen days to a flatter stomach and a younger you ... would you like to have a bikini body without opting out of the real world? You can and you will.' The book says that Stossier believes 90 per cent of us are 'wandering around with irritated intestines' and we should learn to eat properly to cure this and the diseases it causes.

✳ The facts

Much of the advice is a bit like what your grannie used to tell you when you went round to her home for tea – eat slowly, chew thoroughly, don't snack, don't eat sweets …. sort of thing. However I can't agree with the statement that following this regime allows you not to have to opt out of the real world. Whether or not most of us have irritated intestines is something that we will never know.

✳ Health and safety

There is nothing wrong with the foods in the programme – it's an ideal whole, natural and healthy diet, not far removed from standard healthy eating recommendations to cut back on saturates, total fat, salt, sugar, refined foods and so on.

✳ Conclusion

I didn't put this in the detox section because of the claims on the back of the book which seem to turn it into a slimming book, but it is a better option than all the other detox diets mentioned above. If it weren't for the bits of pseudoscience dotted rather frequently throughout the book explaining 'why it works', I would quite like this programme for its emphasis on whole foods, no sugar, proper meals and encouraging mostly sensible eating habits, such as thorough chewing and plenty of decent liquids to drink. Sadly, as it is though, I'm less keen than I should have been – there are too many things you have to do for no seemingly logical reasons.

DIQ: ★★★

The Flat Belly Diet, Liz Vaccariello and Cynthia Sass (Rodale, 2009)

✳ What it is

The book, written by journalists from the US *Prevention* magazine, is based on a study published in the journal *Diabetes Care* in 2007, which found that a diet rich in monounsaturated fatty acids (MUFAs) helped prevent weight gain around the tummy.

✳ The claims

A breakthrough diet for weight loss and belly fat. The diet is rich in MUFAs – the type of fat found in greatest quantity in olive oil, avocados and most nuts and seeds. It also avoids, or is low in, salt, processed foods, wheat-based carbs, fried and spicy foods, fizzy drinks and caffeine and comes with mind tricks to help you beat comfort eating.

✱ The facts

Unfortunately, this is yet another diet book based on a study which turns out to be very small – it was carried out in Spain on only eleven insulin-resistant people and thus any results about the link between MUFAs and reduced belly fat cannot be conclusive. Much more research needs to be done. But it is nice to find a diet reasonably high in good fats – it makes the meals interesting and tasty. It reduces calories, offers satiety and reduces salt and refined foods – almost exactly the same principles as the diet I produced back in 1991, for a book called *A Flat Stomach in 15 Days*!

✱ Health and safety

MUFAs are associated with increased 'good' and lowered 'bad' blood cholesterol, which may protect against heart disease, and the overall diet is varied and healthy enough.

✱ Conclusion

This diet would be OK if it didn't boast a weight loss of 6.8kg (15lb) in a month on a diet of 1600 calories a day – for most overweight women who want to lose 6.3kg (1 stone) or so, that weight loss on such a relatively high calorie level (for slimming) would be very unlikely. It is also a pity there is not more research to back up the premise behind this book.

DIQ: ★★★↲

Raw-food diet

✱ What it is

You eat a diet based on raw plant foods, such as fresh and dried fruits, juices, vegetables, nuts and seeds, sprouted grains and seeds. While some people eat everything raw, others include small proportions of cooked foods, such as fish, grains and pulses.

✱ The claims

Many proponents (among them, actress Demi Moore) believe that plant enzymes important for health and detoxifying the body are lost in cooking, along with vitamins and minerals.

✱ The facts
Research shows that people who follow a raw-plant diet are slimmer than other groups of people because their energy intake is lower. There is also evidence to suggest that eating raw foods speeds up dietary-induced thermogenesis (DIT, see p. 70) and therefore increases your metabolic rate. While some vitamins, such as B and C, can be lost in cooking, a range of vitamins, minerals and plant chemicals, such as beta-carotene, are actually better absorbed in the body when cooked.

✱ Health and safety
Interestingly, there has been research that shows that even though raw fooders are slimmer and have less bone density than people on a typical Western diet, they are no more prone to osteoporosis. One reason may be that the diet is high in magnesium, which is important for calcium absorption, and low in animal protein (known to have a detrimental effect on bone minerals).

Despite lacking dietary vitamin D (important for bone maintenance and found mostly in dairy produce which raw fooders tend not to eat), those studied actually had higher vitamin D concentrations in their bodies than those who follow the typical Western diet.

On paper, the raw-food diet looks to be lacking in a range of nutrients, depending on what proportion of the total diet is, in fact, eaten raw. A person who avoids meat, fish, eggs, dairy, for example, could end up with several deficiencies, unless they were extremely careful to replace these in their diet, which would be no easy job.

✱ Conclusion
An easy, if unusual, way to lose weight without counting calories. I tried this diet for a week, just for interest, and lost 1.3kg (3lb), but found it quite hard to produce tempting meals and ring the changes, even though I am a vegetable lover. I also had high levels of flatulence and was forever in the bathroom. Not a diet for the faint-hearted living in the twenty-first century, but you could do worse than take some of the ideas on board. While the faddy element grates, more natural food, more plant food, sounds good to me. It just doesn't *all* have to be raw.

DIQ: ★★★

Alternate-day fasting/ADF diets

✱ What it is
Simple – as the name suggests, you eat one day and fast the next.

✳ *The claims*

As an example from Jon Benson, author of the *Every Other Day Diet*, you:

> … trick the body into believing calories *are not* being restricted, when in fact *they are.* You do this by cycling your calories. For example, for two days, you eat slightly more calories than your body requires. Then you eat less for two days, more for a single day, and less for two more days. Since the body's metabolism is always kept 'guessing', it never slows down to adapt to a calorie-restrictive diet, and the weight continues to come off …

Other people claim the method helps you lose weight easily without calorie counting, avoids boredom as you only deprive yourself for one day at a time, avoids any potential health problems from actual fasting and can actually increase life span.

✳ *The facts*

The bit about tricking your body/metabolism is more or less nonsense. The metabolism deals with what it is given at any meal/snack occasion; it doesn't think about what you gave it yesterday or wonder what you are going to give it tomorrow.

The success and health of this diet will depend on what you eat on your day off the fast – there are many versions of this diet and some allow almost binge-levels of foods on days off. And the premise that one day you can eat what you want, but the next you need iron willpower may not work for a lot of people. You need to psyche yourself up afresh every other day.

Plus, one day on, one day off may not result in the fat-burning state that's created in loss of appetite, so you could feel very hungry during your fasting days. Lastly, some versions of this diet allow up to 500 calories a day on the 'fasting' days – add that to a binge-type day off and you could actually end up hardly reducing your overall calorie intake enough to result in weight loss. Indeed, 2007 research on mice showed the diet helped prevent weight gain, but didn't achieve weight loss. As I have said before, mice are not men (or women) – so that may not mean a great deal but it does sound logical that such a diet would help a little – but not a lot, as it did for me.

✳ *Health and safety*

The principle behind this idea has been likened to what happens in bulimia, the eating disorder where people binge then purge. The degree of safety and nutritional benefits or drawbacks depends on what you eat on your non-fast day. Also, on fast days you may feel dizzy or have a headache/lethargy.

Although a review of the studies to date published in the *American Journal of Clinical Nutrition* found that small/short research trials on mice showed protection against diabetes, cancer and the risk factors for CHD, there is 'limited human evidence' of benefits (e.g. higher 'good' HDL cholesterol levels and no other results).

✱ *Conclusion*

I tried this way of eating myself for four days and found it unsettling for body, appetite and mind. I didn't lose any weight, as I seemed to feel more hungry for food on the non-fast days. Whether or not this turns out to be OK in health terms, it still smacks too much of high-level faddy eating to me. It teaches nothing about balanced, long-term eating in normal life, and has too many drawbacks to make it a responsible diet.

DIQ: ★

Negative calorie diets

✱ *What it is*

Various books/websites/ebooks claiming that by choosing certain foods over others, you can actually burn off more calories in the digestion of the food, than the food contains, thus creating a 'negative-calorie balance' and weight loss. One ebook, *The Negative Calorie Diet*, whose name is trademarked, from WL publishing, costs $39.90.

✱ *The claims*

> Drop 14 pounds (6.3kg) in 7 days ... a diet plan that results in MASSIVE weight loss ... The digestive system ... processes everything you consume. This process burns calories and results in weight loss! Example: an apple that contains 65 calories may require 100 calories to digest, resulting in a net loss of 35 calories from your body fat. The Negative Calorie Diet identifies over 100 foods that turn your body into a fat-burning machine.

✱ *The facts*

It is quite true that the process of digesting food requires energy – i.e. calories – to perform, and increases our metabolic rate during and after a meal or when something is eaten. As we saw in Chapter Five, protein foods have the most marked effect on the metabolic rate, and the body can use up to 25 per cent of the calories in a protein food during its digestion. But most of the food items in these 'negative calorie' books and diets are vegetables, such as celery and cabbage, or fruits such as apples, high in water and containing virtually no protein.

Yes, foods that are high in fibre (like these) and those which take a longer time to chew and eat are usually those that will result in more energy being used up in their processing. That is why people who follow the raw diet (discussed above) and the vegan diet (all plants, no animal produce) are usually slim – the low calorie content and high energy output to digest these foods keeps people slim. So the negative calorie theory has some truth in it. But, as is often the case, the weight loss benefits are talked up way too much.

✱ Health and safety
If you ate only the 'negative calorie' foods outlined in most of these books you would lose weight quite quickly, but you would also be deficient in various nutrients including protein, several vitamins and minerals.

✱ Conclusion
By all means, eat more raw fruit and vegetables and items that are high in fibre and take a lot of digesting – if your digestive system can take it. (Older people, very young people and people who are ill would all probably be best eating a more easily digested diet.) The book mentioned above is very expensive indeed; if you use your common sense and add lots of low-calorie fresh fruit, salads and vegetables to your diet you will get similar benefits without the considerable financial outlay.

DIQ: ★★↲

DANGER DIETS
While most faddy or quick fix diets can have unwanted side effects, some are downright unhealthy. Here are my Danger Diets … those to avoid.

The Primal Diet
The idea here is that you 'detox' on a diet of 95 per cent raw meat, the fat in which will bind to toxins in your body and help in their removal. The remainder of the diet is vegetable juice, high-fat avocados and a very little dairy, such as rancid yogurt. Eating raw meat (especially, as the diet's deviser Aajonus Vonderplanitz prefers it – aged to the point of rotting) is a huge health risk for

anyone because of the high chance of food poisoning from bacteria in the meat which haven't been killed by cooking, but particularly for the sick and convalescent, the young, the elderly and for pregnant women. Avoid.

Fat Loss For Idiots

'Extremely fast weight loss – lose 9lbs (4.1kg) EVERY 11 days … ' This online downloadable diet book costs $39 and is based on the non-existent principle of 'calorie shifting'. The claim is that 'your body will be given different types of calories each day … which confuses your metabolism and forces FASTER fat loss to happen.' Well, that's nonsense. The diet is a recipe for encouraging eating disorders and psychological damage, and the rate of weight loss is far too high to be healthy for those with an average amount to lose. Avoid.

Fasting

Despite the popular belief that fasting is a good way to 'cleanse the system', prolonged fasts can cause serious harm by depleting protein, calcium, phosphorus, sodium and potassium levels in your body. Fasting can also cause toxic levels of ketones (see p. 110) to build up in the bloodstream. On the other hand, one- to two-day fasts on water, no more than once every few weeks, don't appear to be harmful for healthy people. And it is true that in some areas of the world, fasting is an accepted tradition and people fast for long periods for religious/spiritual reasons and live long lives.

All I can say is – if you want to lead a normal life, stay active, take regular exercise, compete in sport perhaps, maintain muscle mass, avoid high risk of osteoporosis and other ills, get pregnant and so on – then fasting isn't for you. It is also a very dangerous idea for people with previous eating disorders and/or body dysmorphia. Avoid.

The Lemon Detox Diet

I've already analysed this one in detail under the Detox Diets heading (see p. 112), but I'm including it here too.

Note: there are other, general diet habits that can have long-term detrimental effects on your health. For example, a very low-fat diet (where essential fat intake is insufficient) an extremely low-carb diet (where essential dietary fibre is insufficient) and so on. The message: with food intake, extremes of any kind are best avoided.

Moderate Diets

So if you should avoid much of the diet dross that is out there, but you do want some kind of plan to follow, what should you do? There are some diet plans and books which are sensible, healthy and don't rely on pseudoscience, super-fast weight loss or plain nonsense in order to sell. If you want to buy into a plan I suggest one of these:

Stone Age Diet

✱ What it is
A diet based on the food that the hunter-gatherers of the Stone Age used to eat: wild fruit, nuts, seeds, vegetables, wild animals and fish. The book based on this theory – The Paleo Diet by Loren Cordain – was published in 2003 in the USA.

✱ The claims
This is the diet we modern humans forgot how to eat somewhere along the way and if we get back to it, most of our modern ills, including obesity, will disappear.

✱ The facts
The proportions in this diet of the major nutrients – fat, carbohydrates and protein – are very near to the ratio I suggest as an ideal dieting balance in Chapter Five of this book. The carb content is the only major area in which it differs from my recommendations.

✱ Health and safety
Nutrition-wise, you'll get more or less everything you need from this diet if you take a variety from each of the different types of food. It's low on saturates, but with enough unsaturates and omega-3s, and is obviously very, very low in starch, while the overall carb content is not too low, as you get sugars in the fruits. Indeed, the health benefits of a paleo-type diet were analysed in a Swedish scientific study published in July 2009, which concluded that, 'over a three-month study period, a paleolithic diet improved glycaemic control and several cardiovascular risk factors compared to a (standard) diabetes diet in patients with type 2 diabetes'.

✱ Conclusion
I like this diet a lot. It is based on history, rather than bogus science and the foods it contains are healthy, natural, satisfying and naturally calorie-restricting,

so you are likely to lose weight easily. It is almost a stone age Atkins equivalent, without all the fat (wild animals tended to have a very low fat content as do many game birds and animals today) and with no dairy, but more carbs. I also agree with much that the author says about 'how our diet went wrong'.

DIQ: ★★★★✔

The GI Diet

There are very many books that use the glycaemic index (GI) as the basis for a healthy, slimming diet but not all are great. Two of the best are *The GI Diet* by Rick Gallop and *Antony Worrall Thompson's GI Diet*, which has lovely recipes. *The South Beach Diet* is based on low GI, but has a very low-carb start-out programme.

✱ *What it is*
The GI and its significance regarding diet and health is explained more fully on p. 85, but it is basically an index that rates carbohydrate foods on the speed at which they produce blood glucose.

✱ *The claims*
The relevance of GI for slimmers is that low-GI carbs produce a less marked change in blood-sugar levels and may help satiety.

✱ *The facts*
Trying to follow a GI diet can be complicated, as the effect of carbs on blood sugar are also altered by what else is eaten at the same meal – both protein and fat reduce the speed of the GI effect. In fact, all GI diets that work also reduce total energy (calorie) intake.

✱ *Health and safety*
There is increasing debate about the benefits of including a large amount of even low-GI carbs in the diet compared with following a lower-carb diet, such as that outlined in this book. However, generally speaking, low-GI foods (such as pulses, vegetables and some fruits) tend to be those that do have a better all-round health profile than high-GI foods (refined carbs, sugar for example), being usually high in fibre. And, as we know (see the negative calories diet examination, p. 132), they can burn more calories in their digestion than bland, easy-to-swallow/digest, high-GI foods, such as mashed potato and sponge cake.

* Conclusion
Despite ongoing debate about the actual best diet for weight loss/insulin resistance/metabolic syndrome/diabetes and so on (and my feeling that in another ten years' time we may indeed look back at our high complex carb obsession with amusement), the low-GI diets remain some of the best to follow *as things stand*, especially those that include plenty of lean protein and good fats.
DIQ: ★★★★

The Total Wellbeing Diet, Dr Manny Noakes (Michael Joseph, book 1, 2005, book 2, 2007)

* What it is
Manny Noakes is a senior research scientist for the Australian CSIRO (Commonwealth Scientific and Industrial Research Organisation) which devised this weight-loss diet as an answer to all the fads. It became a bestseller in Australia in 2005 and later across the world. The book sets out its rationale for a high-protein, low(ish)-fat and low(ish)-carbohydrate diet, then offers a detailed plan and recipes to cover twelve weeks, plus follow-up maintenance.

* The claims
'The weight-loss programme that can actually work – scientifically tested, easy to use, nutritionally balanced.'

* The facts
While higher in protein than many diets, I don't group this with the high-protein Atkins diet as it contains only around 25 per cent fat and from 20–40 per cent carbs. The CSIRO chose this balance after research in the lab and with people and concluded that – for Australians – it was the balance of nutrients that worked best. The recipes are very meat-based (so not great for vegetarians), but the menus are pleasant, look tempting and easy and a weight loss of around 0.5–1kg (18oz–2¼lb) a week is mentioned.

* Health and safety
The balance of nutrients is in line with much recent research published in bona fide medical journals and in *PubMed* online, which have found medical benefits in eating more protein and less carbs while retaining a reasonable fat content in the diet. The diet provides adequate unsaturates and EFAs, the carb content is largely low GI and the protein is from a variety of sources. There are no nutritional shortfalls.

The diet has a high protein content because in their research the CSIRO found that such a diet produced a much better loss of belly fat in women than did a high-carb, low-fat, 17 per cent protein diet, although elsewhere in the book Noakes says: 'There is no such thing as a "best" way to lose weight – only a best way for you. The way our metabolism works can make a difference to which diet will be the most effective for us.'

✱ Conclusion
While the nutrient balance isn't quite the same as the one I arrived at in Chapter Six in this book, it is similar. They chose less fat, which is interesting, as right up front in the book Noakes says, 'Our very low-fat and higher-fat diets [which they tested before writing the book] resulted in equal weight loss, as long as people consumed the same energy (calories). The higher-fat weight-loss diets had a better effect on blood fats than the very low-fat diets.'

I will finish with a quote Noakes gave in a radio interview some while after the book was published: 'I think a good diet depends very much on the country that you're from and the foods that are available.'

DIQ: ★★★★✦

I CAN MAKE YOU THIN, **PAUL MCKENNA (BANTAM PRESS, 2007)**
Interestingly, you could do worse than read this book by the well-known hypnotist Paul McKenna – not for a diet plan (as it doesn't contain one), but for the emotional back-up it provides. It is packed with motivational and practical tips to help you eat well and thus lose weight. Perhaps it should be called, 'I Can Make You Think'?

DIQ: ★★★★

In conclusion, it appears that honest, truthful, sensible and workable diet plans and books are thin on the ground. But there are some. As Manny Noakes sensibly concluded, there is no such thing as *the* best way to lose weight. A lot of it is about individual preference and personal health profile, the country you live in and what is available.

There are now several research trials showing that rather than any particular set-in-stone balance of major nutrients (fat, protein and carbs) for the easiest/greatest weight/fat loss, it is simply – and always – the creation of a negative energy balance that matters.

That said, certain ways of eating do seem to take the pain out of weight loss and weight control, and any book or system that achieves this will help. In addition to weight loss, a good programme will consider overall health benefits and the effect that combinations of major nutrients have on, for example, blood fats and abdominal fat. Thus my recommendations would be the Paleo Diet (see p. 135) or the Total Wellbeing Diet (see p. 137) – even though neither fits in exactly with the nutritional balance as outlined in Chapter Six, they are not far off!

A responsible, realistic weight control programme will also always include advice on increasing your activity levels and improving your fitness.

Now – let's move on and see how we can save you a great deal of money – and disappointment. Let's look at developing your 'wallet IQ'.

8

Wallet IQ

In an unending quest for the perfect body – or, at least, for a better one than that they currently have – women (and, increasingly, men) spend huge amounts of cash on treatments, products, programmes or activities. But do they actually work? Do they do any good at all? Or are they just a waste of money?

In this chapter, I look at numerous aids to slimming or the body beautiful and give my verdict on each of them. And, where appropriate, I suggest what you might do instead to achieve the desired effect for little or even no cost.

Surgery

Surgery to lose weight or body fat, or to reshape certain parts of the body, is on the increase. Figures for the UK show that 35,000 of us have a 'cosmetic' procedure each year, contributing to an industry that's worth more than £1 billion per annum, while NHS obesity surgery rose 40 per cent in just one year, according to figures in 2009. Not only are the numbers increasing sharply, but the nature of the procedures is changing too.

If you read the blurbs from the private clinics that carry out these procedures, you could be forgiven for thinking that a breast reduction, a bottom lift or liposuction on your belly fat, involves only minor surgery. However, any invasive operation or one that involves an anaesthetic or introducing 'foreign' substances into your body should be viewed with caution.

I underwent five operations in one year a few years back (due to skin cancer), after which I knew, without any doubt, that I would never, ever go under the knife for cosmetic, rather than life-saving, reasons.

There are frequent cases of operations that cause long-term problems, and charlatans practising and offering untested, unlicensed procedures. A *Which?* survey in 2009 exposed hard-selling of operations to people who don't really need them, and sales targets taking precedence over safety.

Cosmetic surgery is neither simple nor foolproof – it can, and does, go wrong and ruins lives. Anyone contemplating any operation, however small, should think very carefully.

Are you a suitable case for treatment?

I believe that cosmetic or weight-related surgery should – in most cases – only ever be even *considered* if you are clinically obese with a BMI of over 35 and/or your operation is deemed necessary by your consultant. And by consultant, I don't mean the person at the private cosmetic surgery clinic who will consult with you before agreeing to do your chosen treatment. I mean your own GP and your own health specialist.

If you are clinically obese and have not managed to lose weight with dietary help and counselling, there is only one procedure that could be useful, and that is gastric banding (or sometimes, possibly, a gastric bypass) – see box, p. 142.

If you were obese and are now a reasonable weight, but have been left with awkward, unsightly skinfolds as a result of your weight loss, the surplus skin can be removed via abdominoplasty, which will leave some scars.

The point is that for people who really *need* them, both of these options are available on the NHS, which begs the question: why go private?

✱ *A sagging belly following childbirth*
If you have a sagging belly after having a baby, but are a reasonable weight, this may be caused by the two columns of the abdominal muscles being pulled apart and becoming permanently stretched during pregnancy and is aggravated by overstretched skin in the same area. Neither exercise nor diet will return the muscles or skin exactly to their pre-baby state, so if you have finished having children you may be offered a tummy tuck which tightens the skin and sews the abdominal muscles back together for more or less permanent results.

A NEW YOU?
Thanks to the success of extreme makeover TV programmes, such as *Ten Years Younger* and *Brand New You*, more people (mostly women) are subjecting themselves to what amounts to almost complete body reshaping. It's not unusual for women to spend over £100,000, not only getting back their younger, firmer bodies, but reshaping the bits they've always disliked, from faces to bums, knees, thighs – even ankles and arms.

As the problem is annoying and slightly unsightly, however, as opposed to life-threatening, you are unlikely to be offered this procedure on the NHS.

✽ *Breast reduction*

This procedure may be recommended for women who are a reasonable weight, but who have uncomfortably large breasts (which can cause back pain and may impede certain activities/sports). Again, this can sometimes be obtained on the NHS although waiting time may be long. If your own NHS GP/consultant agrees you should have a reduction, but you don't want to wait and you can afford it, it may be sensible to go ahead with it privately.

✽ *Liposuction*

One of the most popular cosmetic procedures is liposuction or its current reincarnations which are said to be more effective, such as liposculpture or lipolysis. Since its arrival back in the 1990s, hundreds of private clinics have touted 'lipo' as a harmless, easy, quick way to remove pockets of fat. If you are a reasonable weight, but have stubborn areas of fat which neither diet nor exercise

---

GASTRIC BANDING

This procedure – favoured by TV presenter Fern Britton – is rapidly gaining popularity. A silicone band is inserted into the stomach and inflated with saline to shrink the size of the stomach and thus the amount of food you can eat. (Another procedure is stomach bypass, a more invasive operation which works by making your stomach smaller and your digestive system shorter.)

Suitable for: obese people who have tried over time to eat less and lose weight, and failed. Not for anyone with a few kilograms to lose.

Pros: high success rate. Replaces willpower up to a point, although some people liquidise fast food (easier than eating 'lumpy' food with a band in place) and don't lose weight. A bypass works better for such people.

Cons: procedure has risk element, as well as side effects, including nausea and vomiting if you eat too much or too quickly, and social (you won't enjoy dinner parties much any more).

Alternative: with stomach banding you simply can't overeat without discomfort, so you don't. Nothing else can quite create that effect long term, but some products claim to help you restrict the amount you eat naturally, including the Diet Plate (see below), and therapy (such as CBT or hypnotism) might have a similar effect for some.

will shift (such as saddlebags), many people will probably recommend you try some form of targeted fat removal. Private clinics often make light of the side effects (pain, bruising, swelling), the fact that you have to wear a tight corset for a couple of weeks or so afterwards, possible complications (uneven results, for example) and the fact that while fat cells are removed in the treated area, it is still possible to regain fat, which may appear in other parts of the body.

If you are actually obese, or even fat, lipo isn't the answer, as it works only on 'areas', not your whole body. It's also very expensive – prices start around £2500 but you could easily spend £10,000.

My conclusion on lipo? Rarely necessary – but if you're determined to do it, be aware it isn't for the faint hearted.

So should you opt for surgery?

To summarise:

- Cosmetic and weight-loss surgical procedures range from expensive to eye-wateringly expensive.
- Most cosmetic procedures carried out privately are unnecessary.
- With few exceptions, the results last only a finite period of time – reductions (e.g. breast) being a typical example – nor are they guaranteed to be what you want.
- Things can and do go wrong, regularly.

The only winners in the long term are the clinics and surgeons who make a very good living on our insecurities.

If you do have money to burn, consider spending it on exercise equipment (see Chapter Nine), regular relaxing and life-affirming activity holidays, setting yourself up in business, giving it to your kids, putting it into a retirement fund ... there are lots of ways to spend a lot of money which can give as much or more pleasure than surgery and which may be of more use.

Diet Pills

Take a pill and lose weight without having to do much else – sounds great, which is why in the UK we spend £50 million on over-the-counter pills every year and the NHS spend many millions more, with 1.06 million prescriptions being dispensed for the treatment of obesity.

Prescription slimming pills

✱ *Orlistat (brand name Xenical)*
This works by preventing the body from absorbing fats from the diet, which should result in weight loss. At the standard dose of 120mg, three times a day, orlistat prevents approximately 30 per cent of dietary fat from being absorbed.

Since April 2009, orlistat has been available over the counter at chemist shops in the UK at half strength (60mg dose) under the brand name Alli. At this dose, the drug prevents absorption of around 25 per cent of dietary fat.

Pharmacists must weigh customers before they can sell them the pill and it should, in theory, only be used by adults with a BMI of 28 or more, though reports suggest people weighing less than this have been able to purchase it with no problems. GlaxoSmithKline, manufacturers of the drug, say that clinical trials show that 'adding orlistat to a reduced-calorie, lower-fat diet, can help people lose 50 per cent more weight than dieting alone'.

People taking the drug are advised to avoid fatty foods and stick to a reduced-calorie diet, so it isn't the easy option you might think. If you continue to eat a high-fat diet, there are frequent side effects, such as diarrhoea, oily stools and even actual liquid fat leakage.

Year-long clinical trials of orlistat showed up to half of people achieved a 5 per cent plus weight loss. As an example, for someone who at 1.65m (5ft 5in) tall, weighing in at 82.5kg (13 stone) has a BMI of 31, this represents a weight loss of 4.1kg (9lb) plus – not a great deal over a year.

Also, after orlistat was stopped, a significant number of people gained weight – up to 35 per cent of what they had lost. Lastly, one Norwegian study found that people who had been on orlistat for a year ended up eating more fat than people who were not on the drug.

Professor Gareth Williams of Bristol University has said that people on Alli reduce their calorie intake only 100 calories a day more than if they just did the diet and exercise and didn't take the pills.

Alli is not a cheap option, either. So for people determined to try orlistat it would be more sensible to see their GP, get a prescription for a month's supply for a fraction of the cost and get double strength.

My view is that because of possible side effects, the fact you have to diet anyway and the relatively insignificant weight loss and long-term benefits, I would not join the 30 million people worldwide who have tried Xenical in the past ten years.

✱ *Sibutramine (brand name Reductil)*
This can help to speed up weight loss, both by suppressing appetite and increasing the metabolic rate. It should only be used under strict medical supervision and in conjunction with diet and exercise measures. It's only suitable for people with a BMI of more than 30 or for people with a BMI of more than 27 who also have other health problems, such as diabetes or high blood cholesterol. Side effects include increased blood pressure, headaches, dry mouth, constipation, insomnia, itchy nose, sore throat and increased heart rate.

✱ *Prescription slimming pills – conclusion*
Prescription slimming pills may be useful for some people, particularly those with severe obesity who have tried and failed to lose weight by other means and who have been advised by their doctor to try them.

But for the rest of us, here's a cautionary tale to end on. Back in 2006, a new, prescription slimming pill was launched on the UK market (and other areas). Called rimonabant (brand name Acomplia), it was shown to work by reducing appetite. By 2008, the drug was available in fifty-six countries, but in October of that year, the European Committee for Medicinal Products for Human Use (CHMP) concluded that the benefits of Acomplia no longer outweighed its risks (of depression, serious psychiatric disorders and even suicide). Manufacturers Sanofi-Aventis later suspended the drug and it is unlikely ever to be manufactured or sold again.

The moral? Just because something has been trialled and approved by all the right official bodies and you are handed a prescription by your doctor, does not necessarily mean it is safe. As prescription pills (and Alli) are, at best, only partially successful in helping people to lose weight and keep it off, and none is without side effects, I recommend that they are only ever used as a very last resort. As the wise Professor Gareth Williams, obesity expert and author of *Obesity: Science to Practice*, says: 'The dent [a drug like Alli] makes on your life and health is very small. We should be pedestrianising cities, building cycle tracks, getting people moving – not dumping all the responsibility on to a drug.'

Supplements

So you haven't tried prescription pills – but I bet you have, somewhere in your home, a bottle of half-used supplements which you bought in your local 'health food' shop, chemist or online because of the hype about their role in helping you to slim.

Here are some of the likely contenders:

✱ Fat magnets

Claims: they block fat in the diet from being absorbed in the body. They often contain chitosan – a derivative of ground shell from shellfish – which Harvard University in the USA says you should not buy because it is ineffective. Other studies have shown limited fat-blocking effects but the number of pills you'd need to take for any real effect is much more than the recommended dose.

Brands: many (over 100 million have been sold to date), mostly calling themselves simply Fat Magnets, or Fat Magnets Plus.

Cost: around £20 for 120 pills, 4–6 a day recommended. Other types of fat-blocker are also widely available, based on products such as ficus – a cactus derivative.

Conclusion: a high-calcium, moderate-fat diet would be a better and cheaper alternative. There is also a worry that if these did work, essential omega fats may be blocked – many of us don't get enough of these in our diets and this could be a real health problem. Fat-soluble vitamin absorption could also be affected and a study showed that mineral absorption and bone density are reduced in animals fed chitosan.

✱ Starch-blockers

Claims: they contain a substance called phaseolamin which is said to stop starch in food from being absorbed – so you can eat bread, potatoes, cakes, biscuits and lose weight. 'Neutralise up to a third of your calories!' says one internet banner.

Brands: many, with names such as carb-slim, starch-blocker phase 2.

Cost: around £35 for a three-week supply (up to eight pills a day) is typical.

Conclusion: starch-blockers have been around since the 1980s. Over ten years ago one of the UK's leading obesity experts, Professor John Garrow, said:

> 'There is an element of truth in these claims: phaseolamin can be extracted from beans which, when mixed in a test tube with amylase (the enzyme which normally digests starch in the small bowel) inactivates the enzyme. The untrue part [is] that by eating phaseolamin you could stop the absorption of the calories in your diet. The reason is that phaseolamin is itself a protein, so the protein-digesting enzymes in the stomach break it up into amino acids. By the time it gets into the small bowel, where starch digestion takes place, the phaseolamin has itself been digested, and has no effect on starch digestion.'

In recent years, more research has been done on the effects of phaseolamin in the body and found that a prescription version may help diabetics to reduce their insulin medication. But still, most studies to date show no or only slight weight loss and official advice is over-the-counter versions aren't worth buying. On a safety level – starch-blocker pills may be toxic because they contain raw beans. Side effects of the pills can be wind and bloating.

I also have an ethical objection to both starch blockers and fat magnets: while the world debates how to secure food for the whole population in years to come, how can we justify eating food if it isn't going to be absorbed?

A much better alternative is to follow the dietary suggestions outlined in Chapter Six; reducing your carb intake naturally and eating more 'good carbs' will help you lose weight – and not cost money.

Herbal products

* Appesat

This works by tricking the brain into thinking the stomach is full. You take three pills, made from seaweed extract, with a large glass of water at least half an hour before meals, and as they swell in your stomach, they stimulate receptors to signal the brain that you're full. At £29.95 for a pack of fifty (and nine a day recommended for the first three weeks), it is expensive, but it is an approved medical device assessed under the European Medical Devices Directive. Should work for steady weight loss for people who are overweight through over-large meals rather than, say, mindless snacking.

* Spirulina

This is a type of algae found in lakes which is used as fish food as it is rich in trace nutrients – it is sometimes marketed as helping to control food cravings, but Harvard University has found it ineffective.

* Hoodia

This is a South African plant said to help suppress appetite, but trials on humans are limited and show mixed results. A look at discussion boards shows that people who have tried it are by and large not very impressed with the results; one problem may be that the active ingredient, dubbed P57, may not be present in many of the pills sold as hoodia.

* Ephedra (ma huang)

This is a natural form of ephedrine which increases metabolic rate and dulls appetite. Ephedra has been banned in the USA since 2004 and is also illegal in the UK as a supplement, as it has a high risk factor for heart attack – ironic as it is one of the few supplements known to work, at least for the first few months. Forms of ephedra are still available on the internet in many diet pills, such as 'bitter orange' (*citrus orantium*), which has been declared unsafe by Harvard, and country mallow – both of which contain ephedra-like chemicals. Best avoided.

* Zotrim

This contains South American plant extracts yerbe mate, damiana and caffeine-rich guarana. The pills are said to make you feel fuller quicker, keeping appetite at bay, as well as increasing energy and helping to burn calories. It has undergone clinical trials which show moderate results in helping weight loss and maintenance, but the manufacturer's website advocates normal 'eat less and exercise more' advice alongside. At approximately £21.50 for a month's supply, it is less expensive than many, but the modest results could, I feel, be obtained simply through diet and exercise.

* Herbal products – conclusion

There are many herbal pills that are said to help weight loss, the above being just a few of the better-known ones, and I can safely say that most will empty your purse faster than your fat cells.

A less expensive and truly natural alternative to herbal products is to use natural foods – such as lean protein, raw foods and spices – to help boost metabolism (see p. 99).

Diuretics and laxatives

Neither diuretics (pills to increase the amount of urine you excrete) nor laxatives (which speed up the passage of food through the digestive system, colon and bowel) should be used as aids to slimming. Regular use of diuretics can flush minerals from the body, while regular use of laxatives can cause dependence and malabsorption of nutrients (and, used frequently, can actually make constipation worse). In any case, diuretics won't produce fat loss, only fluid loss, and laxatives will only produce marginal weight loss as the passage of food is speeded up. Best avoided. Instead, drink more water and eat plenty of high-fibre, low-calorie vegetables.

Metabolism-boosters

These are supposed to speed up the rate at which your body burns the calories you eat and drink. As we've seen in Chapter Five, several types of food can increase metabolic rate – protein foods, coffee and green/white tea being examples. Caffeine and green tea are frequently listed in the ingredients for metabolism-boosting pills, but often the amounts contained in the pills are unlikely to achieve much. Many pills contain a long list of ingredients, including items such as ginseng, kola nut, bladderwrack, garcinia, chromium which are unlikely to be of more than peripheral use. A regular cup of green tea would be much cheaper and probably more effective.

The diet outlined on p. 95 will help boost metabolism, as will regular activity.

Others

There is a huge variety of different diet pill ingredients on the market and not enough room here to analyse them all – from HGH (Human Growth Hormone) through creatine, L-carnitine and L-tyrosine (amino acids) to DHEA (an energy-boosting hormone) and dozens more. You could spend a fortune and lose no pounds except those in your purse. Plus, many may have unwanted or potentially dangerous side effects.

Diet pills – conclusions

Unlicensed pills and potions for weight loss are classed as food supplements and controlled by food regulations. As such, they are not required to go through proper scientific testing before being put on sale, as long as they don't make direct health or therapeutic claims on the pack. As for what is classified as a health claim and what is not, this is a grey area, hence you'll see phrases like, 'Eat all the foods you love and still lose weight!', 'Fire your body's fat-burning furnace!' or 'Feel full without eating less!'

Some of the pills may have a temporary positive effect, but this could be due to the placebo effect – you want it to work and you unconsciously reduce your food intake or adjust your eating habits while you take the pills. Indeed, this theory has been tested for a month, during which 70 per cent of the people taking placebo pills lost weight: a success story indeed.

Diet Products

Slimming drinks

Why pay £1.50 for fifty tea bags which may help you lose weight when you can pay £37.49 for sixty? That's what I wonder when I look at the hundreds of websites selling slimming teas such as *Pu-erh*, the one said to be favoured by Victoria Beckham. The research for this particular tea shows no benefits for weight loss over ordinary green tea (see p. 91) and indeed any weight loss effects could simply be due to the fact that drinkers give up the milk (and possibly sugar) when they swap from ordinary tea or coffee. But some sites really are charging £37.49 including postage and packing for sixty bags.

Then there is Coffee Slender – an instant coffee containing a decaffeinated green coffee extract Svetol, which in one small trial showed promising results for weight loss and helps regulate blood-sugar levels which could reduce cravings. Svetol contains chlorogenic acids which are said to be the main active ingredient. This may well be the case, but more research needs to be done. The product is not harmful as a coffee replacement and is low in caffeine, but is very pricey (at about £12.95 for twenty-one sachets). Whether the benefits over standard coffee are worth that, I am not sure. For more on coffee, see p. 91.

Slimatee is basically a laxative, containing senna and a few other plant derivatives. As, we've seen above, laxatives should not be used for slimming.

Slimming patches, pens and other gimmicks

In 2008, the Advertising Standards Authority banned a TV ad by the 'Pink Patch' as it said there was no evidence the ingredients (such as fucus and 5-HTP) in the patch caused any weight loss. Nevertheless, the patch is widely sold on the internet (at £35.95 plus postage and packing, for one month's supply). And

---

THE INTERNET

Although you can find bogus slimming products at your local chemist or health store, they are mostly sold on the internet. Be very careful what you believe when you visit slimming sites. I've just looked at one – as an example – that claims to analyse the top twenty slimming pills, but each has a link to the site selling these products, meaning that the analysis is far from unbiased.

It's also a good idea to download a good spam-blocker to bar unwanted emails that are trying to sell you products.

there are dozens of other 'slimming patches' to be found. My advice is to take the ASA's line and ignore these products.

And the same goes for pens that you sniff to help you lose weight, the diet hand cream that contains green tea and the 'detox' foot patches that will help you slim and fight off illness. All of this is available on a website called Slimming Solutions – one of the worst I've seen for peddling overpriced nonsense.

The Diet Plate

A fairly simple way to help portion control, this is a normal dinner plate divided into painted sections for carbs, protein, vegetables, pasta and sauces. There's also a cereal/soup bowl. My only objection is the price – from the official website the plate is a whopping £24 (including postage and packing) and the bowl not much less. I know of people this has helped, but of course it won't help with finger foods, snacks on the run, drinks and so on.

DIY Cellulite Treatments

Cellulite is the orange-peel-like fat many women (even slim ones) carry just under the skin on their lower bodies. The cause seems to be that women's subcutaneous fat cells are held in place in sacs between fibrous connective tissue. Because these fibres can't expand, fluctuating weight, pregnancy or simply time can cause the fat globules to distort and create the dimpled effect which can be accentuated by fluid retention and ageing skin.

Cellulite creams, which are massaged into your dimpled skin, are many and mostly expensive – some as much as £100. An overview of all the tests on real people that I can find seems to show that they are 95 per cent a waste of time – if there is any difference in cellulite after using them regularly for weeks, it is small, and inch loss is similarly small or non-existent.

In fact, as most women who use the creams tend also to change their eating habits and/or exercise habits while using them, it's nearly impossible to say whether the creams have any effect at all, other than making the surface of the skin smoother (but that is likely to be down to the massage or body brushing that's usually advised).

Exercise is the best treatment for cellulite (take a look – if they'll let you! – at the legs, hips and bums of professional athletes and I doubt you'll find any cellulite on them at all), coupled with an ordinary moisturiser smoothed or massaged into the skin, if you like. A healthy diet with plenty of lean protein and essential fats will also help – as will a bit of fake tan.

DIY Body Wraps

DIY body wraps for 'inch loss' are sold at around £7–10 each (which is cheap, compared with salon treatments) and they do work to help shed inches temporarily from the stomach, thighs or bottom, for example, for a quick fix when you need to get into that party dress. But they can be messy to apply and awkward to use (I know – I tried one myself). A pack usually comprises bandages (or similar), sachets of clay-mix combined with ingredients said to draw out toxins. For example the 'Wrap Factor' cream contains 'a fusion of natural ingredients – almond oil, vitamin E, fennel, juniper berry and cypress – that work in harmony with each other and with your body, to leave you feeling refreshed, invigorated and purified. Firm, tone, detox and lose inches in one simple process.'

But you can't 'firm and tone' fat (which is what cellulite is) – you can only firm and tone muscle (which it isn't). The inch reduction is simply displaced fluid and the compression effect from the bandages, and it will soon return whatever the website or blurb tells you to the contrary. And there is no way that a clay pack can draw toxins from your fat cells via your skin (and even if it could it would make no difference at all to your body-fat percentage).

To achieve the body-wrap effect (without the body wrap), cut back hard on carbs before a special event – this will keep you going to the loo and reduce your body's water content significantly, particularly noticeably around the abdomen. Or try some magic knickers – much less bother and you don't need to keep buying new ones.

Salon/Clinic Treatments

If you don't fancy DIY creams or wraps, you can go to a 'beauty' salon and pay several times as much (from £45–125, depending on the salon and treatment) for more or less the same thing. A typical promise is for around 15cm (6in) lost in one session, but what they don't tell you is that this figure is the total loss in several different body parts (even including the wrist and forearm).

You can also get your wobbly bits attacked by some form of electrical stimulation, powerful rollers or suction effect. Of these, I can find only one which has a proper seal of approval. This is Endermologie, which was licensed by the

US Food and Drug Administration as having a temporary effect on improving the appearance of cellulite through a combination of motorised roller massage and suction. This increases circulation to the area massaged – i.e. blood and oxygen – and encourages lymphatic drainage of fluid and waste products. The deep manipulation also helps stimulate and stretch connective tissue.

A single session of Endermologie costs between £50 and £60, but to get the full benefit, salons recommend a course of fourteen to twenty-eight sessions (from around £650), for two to three sessions a week, at least in the beginning. Then you'll need maintenance sessions once or twice a month to maintain the effects. And, surprise, surprise – it works best on people who are no more than 12.7kg (2 stone) overweight, who exercise regularly and eat a healthy diet.

Conclusion

If you've money to burn, Endermologie is worth a try. Do remember, however, that no matter how much your body fat/cellulite are mobilised, unless you exercise or eat less to burn off the mobilised fat calories, they will simply settle back into those comfy fat cells once again.

It's also worth noting that trials done on people to test the efficacy of any of the above products or treatments have been small; most are not proper clinical trials and results – especially with inch loss – are easy to manipulate. Furthermore, testimonials from satisfied clients – especially on the internet – are often made up, while chat rooms are invaded by 'interested parties' posing as punters, to big up the products.

So be very discriminating when reading any reports and recommendations.

Other Treatments

Massage

Normal, manual, deep-tissue Swedish-type massage may be almost as good at draining the lymph glands and creating water loss as the treatments described above – after any good massage you will find yourself needing to go to the loo for that reason. But massage isn't cheap, and once again, you're not losing fat.

Acupuncture

I can find little evidence that acupuncture helps weight loss. There are cases of people who have acupuncture and lose weight, but this may be because, for example, their stress levels are reduced and therefore comfort eating is reduced too. A recent overview of acupuncture trials used for various health problems, published in 2009, also found that fake acupuncture worked just as well as real acupuncture – i.e. it is that placebo effect at work again.

Hypnotism

You may be surprised, but I do think that hypnotism can be helpful as a weight-loss tool. A good hypnotist will retrain your mind to create the willingness to change your lifestyle habits, i.e. what you eat and the exercise you do. It can also alter your relationship with food, say from fearing it to enjoying it. Two or three sessions should be enough to achieve results so it's worth a try (from £90 an hour – the industry is unregulated, so to find a decent practitioner, check on www.ukcho.co.uk).

BODY FAT MONITORS/SCALES

You can pay a lot of money (up to £200) for home scales which tell you how much body fat you're carrying, as well as your weight and perhaps even your water content. Most of them work by sending a 'bioelectrical impedance' signal through the body which passes freely through muscle and bone, but encounters resistance when passing through fatty tissue.

These might be useful if you're borderline overweight or want to check if your weight is mostly fat or muscle. The disadvantage is that they don't tell you whether your fat is mostly in your belly (so a health risk) or elsewhere (less of a health risk).

The waist circumference test (see p. 44) or even looking in the mirror naked should be able to tell you whether you're carrying to much fat around your middle without costing a penny.

Slimming Clinics

Private slimming clinics exist in just about every major town and city in the UK and most offer a combination of dietary advice (the quality of which varies) and prescription slimming pills. Prices range from a reasonable £16 a week for the advice and prescription (Weight Medics) up to £99 for a three-day diet diary analysis and forty-five minute phone or personal consultation with a nutritionist (National Nutrition Clinic) or more.

If clinics aren't medication-based they may sell other costly procedures. Food intolerance testing is frequently offered (intolerance often being cited as a reason for weight problems), using methods such as Vega (electromagnetic) or hair analysis, which are known to produce poor results and cost from around £50 up to £300. As Dr Adrian Morris, allergy specialist at the London Medical Centre, says: 'Clinical studies have repeatedly shown Vega testing to be ineffective in diagnosing allergies and intolerances.'

Conclusion

Anything of any use that you would get at most slimming clinics, you should be able to get for free – or for the price of a prescription – at an NHS surgery, if you are truly in need of it. Your GP should be able to offer you dietary advice or refer you to a local dietician and will prescribe slimming pills, if appropriate. If not, you shouldn't be getting the pills privately, anyway. Many clinics aren't regulated in any way and some offer dubious dietary or other advice or procedures. Most people would be better off buying a decent book on nutrition and going to a slimming club or similar for support.

Spas

While there are not many full-blown spas (which used to be called 'health farms') in the UK, all-inclusive trips to foreign spas are gaining popularity. A spa may give you a chance to get your mind and body in gear to begin a healthier lifestyle. But if the 'health holiday' is to be worth the money, you need to choose a spa that fits in with your needs, which isn't that easy, as they vary in almost every way. You can get luxury or spartan, severe or relaxed diet, lots of beauty treatments or none, good or poor exercise facilities and so on.

Conclusion

Spas are expensive, but the kick-start may be helpful. But if you just want a rest, a light diet, some beauty treatments and a swimming pool, it may be less expensive simply to book a hotel with a salon and pool (though you'll need some willpower to choose the healthier meals from the menu). And if you simply want to get slimmer, a walking holiday would be even better and much cheaper.

Boot Camps

If you don't mind working out twelve hours a day, getting down and dirty in places like the mountains of mid-Wales and being shouted at, you might like one of the new breed of boot camps, designed especially for unfit, overweight civilians. You go for a week and by the end you can see your toes again and even touch them.

The level of (dis)comfort and the amount and quality of food, exercise and accommodation varies from camp to camp, but two of the best-reviewed are GI Jane and New You. (New You even do a luxury version – instead of staying in a bunk bed in a dorm, you stay in a comfortable room in a country-house hotel!) Needless to say, the word 'camp' belies the cost; these courses aren't inexpensive and you won't see much, if any, change from £1000 for a week.

Conclusion

Could be a good idea for a kick-start if you have residual levels of fitness and enjoy a challenge. If you are extremely unfit and very overweight, I would think twice before taking a boot camp on because, by their nature, these programmes are tough – and as we will see in the next chapter, unfit, overweight people are safer beginning to exercise gently. Also, trying to measure up against the people on the course who ARE fit could hit already-low self esteem.

My advice is to maybe do the spa this year and try it next year when you've lost a bit of weight and won't have to stress in case you're the last person chosen for the bootcamp team.

Slimming Clubs

There is proper published evidence to suggest that attending a slimming club makes the business of weight loss easier, and there is also evidence that people who keep the weight off are over twice as likely to have been part of a group. This could be for several reasons:

- the motivation of being weighed (if the particular club does that – not all do)
- the support of other people in 'the same boat'
- the support of a leader, adviser or counsellor who has probably lost weight too

- a designated eating plan – perhaps with exercise advice or, in one or two cases, participation, too (most meeting halls don't have facilities for everyone to exercise)

Clubs are generally not too expensive and there are plenty scattered across the country, so you don't usually have to trek miles to find one. There is also usually an online membership option. Once you've reached your desired weight, there is long-term support – usually you can attend the meetings on an occasional basis.

All in all, a good idea for most of us. However, not everyone likes what can sometimes feel like the 'back to school' atmosphere of attending a class/meeting. Also, some leaders are better than others (they are not usually professionally qualified, but trained by the clubs themselves) and each club follows a different eating plan.

WeightWatchers

WeightWatchers is, perhaps, the best-known slimming club, having been around since 1963 (started in the States). It relies on a points system which, to my mind, is the only drawback, as it's just another way of counting calories and saturated fats, and seems to make things more complicated, not less. However, this is a small gripe.

WeightWatchers' 2009 Discover Plan helps members choose healthy and filling options. WW are reliably good and affordable at a cost of £9 to join and a weekly fee of about £5.50. All that said, I emailed their press office twice for more detailed information on their programme and received only a short, uninformative reply.

Slimming World

Slimming World was founded in 1969. It operates a 'food optimising' system that gives you 'free foods' (no weighing or measuring), healthy extras that need weighing, and 'syns' – items they consider to be 'naughty extras' (these used to be called 'sins' – but the 'y' doesn't fool me!). I don't like the syns idea, it makes me feel uneasy, but I guess it works for the members. It costs £10 to join and a weekly fee of £4.50.

Rosemary Conley Diet and Fitness Clubs

These were founded in 1993 and are the only major clubs that offer a proper full-length exercise class with qualified (Oxford, Cambridge and Royal Society of

LOOK GOOD FOR LESS

Here are five cost-free ways to help you look good:

- **Get a good night's sleep.** Research shows that sleep deprivation causes increased body weight because it reduces levels of the protein leptin in the body, which regulates body fat, and increases levels of ghrelin, which stimulates appetite. Good sleep may also increase your energy levels and improve mood, both of which can positively influence food choices and exercise output.

- **Tum the central heating down.** Over the years, the average temperature in our homes has increased, but our bodies burns more calories in a cool atmosphere rather than a warm one. Of course, this will also save you money!

- **Only take medication that is really necessary.** Many types of medicines, including antidepressants, sleeping pills, high blood pressure pills, beta-blockers, contraceptives and others can make you more prone to weight gain.

- **Lead a natural life.** There is some evidence that some pesticides that are used widely for food and clothing production and chemicals used in some plastics for food packaging can cause hormonal disturbances which may make you more prone to weight gain.

- **Alternative alarm call.** Every year we spend more and more of our leisure time in sedentary activities, including computer use and watching TV. Reduce this by thirty minutes a day (set an alarm to go off, so you don't forget), and use that time to do something physically active. On average, this could result in expending an extra 6.3 kilogram's worth (1 stone) of calories a year.

Arts/OCR) instructors in exercise to music, who also have an accredited certificate in applied nutrition and weight management – a big plus point for me. Members currently receive a copy of Conley's *GI Hip and Thigh Diet* which is a low-fat, low-GI diet as their main tool for losing weight; other than that there is simply a five-minute motivational talk and a weigh-in. The cost is £10 to join and weekly fees vary by area.

Online diet clubs

All the above offer online support which varies in detail and cost. There are also various dedicated online slimming organisations and programmes, such as Tesco Diets (various membership plans, costing on average £2 a week) and Weight Loss Resources (£9.74 a month). Both offer regular support, tailored healthy diet plans and a range of other resources, including recipes, background information, member forums and news. For anyone who prefers not to go to a club, I think either of these is good, though my favourite is WLR.

Conclusion

Of everything listed in this chapter, clubs are one of the least expensive options and the most likely to be helpful, in my opinion.

In conclusion, we all sometimes feel we 'deserve' special treatments, spas, consultations and so on. We want to be pampered, to feel loved, special, important or even just simply given attention and to be noticed. If people in our normal lives aren't doing that or if life is dull, then often, we'll pay. And, in such cases, the weight loss or body improvements are almost immaterial – an unimportant (albeit welcome) by-product. So if you want pampering – that's fine, pay for luxury massages or a spa weekend and enjoy it.

But the fact is that looking good, staying a reasonable weight and feeling good do not *need* to cost a lot of money. You would be much better off splashing out on some nicely cut underwear or clothes, a good haircut or even the services of a personal trainer.

On analysis, the perceived benefits of what we've looked at in this chapter are as follows:

1. **The quick-fix factor**: weight loss (supposedly) for little or no effort (through surgery, slimming pills, wraps) which appeals to the lazy side of all of us.
2. **Support**: through clinic attendance, slimming clubs – we don't want to do it on our own, especially if we've failed before.
3. **Scientific validation**: through allergy testing, for example – can validate your previous inability to lose weight and kick-start renewed efforts.
4. **Motivation**: a quick start at a spa or boot camp or the promise of a 'gold star' at a slimming club – this works in all areas of life, including (at least temporarily) weight control.
5. **Hope**: the promise of a cure via hypnotism or by joining a group – a vital factor in making a new start.

In the remainder of the book, I intend to offer, if not quick-fix ideas, then certainly alternative suggestions to give you support, validation, motivation and hope.

Part Three:
The Escape

9
Fitness IQ

Exercise is good. We all know that. Yet despite knowing we should exercise, many of us fail to do so, and I believe there are two reasons for this:

1. We don't *need* to exercise to live our everyday lives.
2. We don't *want* to exercise – we don't see it as either enjoyable or life-enhancing.

So it stands to reason – if you don't need to do it and you don't want to do it, why on earth bother?

But before we go any further, for all us exercise haters, I have some pleasant news ....

You don't actually have to do that much.

We all know the friend who exercises three hours a day, every day, rain or shine. The celeb who works out with a personal trainer five hours a day. We read about the elite athletes who get up at 5 a.m. and train all day and forgo a social life for their sport. Because we feel daunted by the thought of a lot of exercise, instead of doing just a little – we do none. In the UK, only 37 per cent of men and 24 per cent of women take enough exercise to get any benefit from it.

Ironically, when it comes to exercise, it's rarely the case that the more you do, the better the outcome. For most of us who aren't professional sportspeople, enough is enough, and more than enough may well be too much (see box, p. 165).

For general wellbeing and health protection (e.g. to cut risk of heart disease by 50 per cent), the Department of Health suggests half an hour's moderate-intensity aerobic activity five times a week. For help with weight loss this goes up to an hour five days a week. The World Health Organisation and the UK Fitness Industry Association also recommend 30 x 5, while the USA's Center for Disease Control and Prevention's latest 2008 guidelines are 2½ hours of moderate OR 1¼ hours of vigorous exercise a week OR a combination of the moderate and vigorous exercise goals PLUS two weekly sessions of resistance (weight) training to maintain muscle strength and bone density.

But recently, researchers at Queen's University, Belfast, found walking for half an hour just three days a week gave similar fitness and blood pressure benefits to walking for thirty minutes five times a week. And an Australian study found that people who simply potter around, or stand every time they have the opportunity rather than sitting, are healthier and slimmer than sedentary people. And you need to burn just an extra 150 calories a day through exercise to prevent dangerous build-up of fat around your organs. That's equivalent to no more than fifteen minutes on, for example, a stepping machine.

And at the other end of the scale, the British Association of Sports and Exercise Sciences say that you SHOULDN'T burn up MORE than 3,000 calories in exercise a week – i.e. 600 x 5 days a week. To burn 600 calories you'd need to moderate jog for an hour, fast cycle for 1¼ hous, or walk briskly for about 1¾ hours.

The truth is that there IS no cast iron answer to how much exercise you 'should' do. Just as Body Mass Index is a set of figures plucked out of the bag as a starting point to define obesity, so the exercise amount guidelines are just a guide. Paul Gately, Professor of Exercise and Obesity at Leeds Metropolitan University, says it is very difficult to formulate a 'one size fits all' policy for exercise, as moderate exercise for one would be intense for another. In other words, if you are unfit and unused to exercise, you might start on just five minutes a day and still get benefits from that.

Assuming we are sticking with 'official' recommendations, there have been mutterings within the fitness industry in the UK who have been concerned that these guidelines give a false impression – that all you need is a stroll or a bit of gardening to keep you fit and thus they may encourage us to do even less.

Like the food industry, as we saw earlier in the book, the fitness industry is there to make money – the gym, the classes, the personal training for example – and has a vested interest in ensuring we don't all think a brisk walk is going to do the trick.

Complicated? A thorny subject? Well it needn't be. All you need to know is how much is enough for you – and that may be different from other people's optimum level. To discover this it pays to be able to listen to your body and that way you'll soon discover what is your own fitness IQ – the right line between too much and not enough. (We'll be looking at this in more detail on p. 171.)

What Are Fitness and Exercise?

Fitness usually refers to cardiovascular fitness – i.e. the fitness of your heart and lungs. A fit heart beats more slowly than an unfit heart and fit lungs can take in more air and utilise it more efficiently with each breath than unfit lungs. But true fitness is three-cornered; it also includes muscular strength and joint flexibility.

Exercise is what people do consciously to try to get fit (or fitter), using the physical body – putting it through its full range of movement to increase flexibility, make the heart and lungs work harder to improve stamina and boost muscle strength (known as the stamina/strength/flexibility triangle).

THE DANGERS OF OVER-EXERCISING

Ironically, when it comes to exercise, beyond a certain point, it's rarely the case that the more you do, the better the outcome. For most of us who aren't professional sportspeople, enough is enough, and more than enough may well be too much.

- Exercise can be addictive and create a dependency, much like a drug, because physical activity – particularly vigorous or prolonged – produces endorphins which give you a 'high'. People who over-exercise are often also anorexic.
- Physical injury is common in sportspeople and in ordinary people who do the wrong type of exercise, or the right kind in the wrong way. One report from Australia found that one in five of people trying boot camp-style exercises injured themselves.
- Long-term, high-impact exercise (such as jogging) can cause joint injury, damage to the cartilage of the knees being typical.
- Repetitive exercises, especially if done wrongly, can cause lower back and neck pain.
- Increasing your heart rate outside your safe range may cause a heart attack, and the *American Journal of Cardiology* recently reported that in general, over-exercising can increase the risk of heart problems.
- Over-exercising can lower the immune system, reduce body fat to dangerously low levels and, in women, cause amenorrhoea (lack of periods) and/or later in life, osteoporosis.
- Obese people who do high-impact exercise, such as aerobics or running, are at higher than average risk of joint problems, including arthritis because the extra weight places increased stress on the joints.

Need and Want: How to Achieve Them

If – as we've seen above – not needing and not wanting to exercise are what's standing in our way, let's now look at how we can get past them.

Need

For thousands of years, fitness was achieved quite naturally and we didn't even have to think about it. We used to hunt for food by walking and running many miles each day. We used to move home regularly by walking from clearing to clearing – this would involve climbing hills and mountains, crossing streams. In the farming era we toiled all day to grow crops or tend animals with no power tools, no electricity. Even in the early office years, we walked to talk to colleagues, rather than sending an email or using the phone. We commuted to work, often by walking or cycling, not by car or train. And at home, we used energy scrubbing, polishing, sweeping and cutting grass, whereas now we have power tools for every job.

Now half of kids, a new report says, don't ever go out to play. We're raising a nation of couch/computer potatoes.

With our long-term daily physical challenges gone, we – modern man and woman – have indeed lost the *need* to walk, lift, move, use our bodies. Our entire natural keep-fit programme has gone. What we need now is to *need* exercise once again.

✳ Creating the need

Telling yourself that exercise is good for your health doesn't work well for most of us because the idea is too abstract (although, having said that, I still feel the need to mention the many health benefits on p. 168 because seeing them in writing may induce a need, in some of us, to get on the walking boots).

I believe that much of our inability to maintain activity is because we think of it in terms of 'artificial' exercise – 'Exercise' with a capital E – like an aerobics class or the gym, which is an end in itself, with no purpose other than getting fit. And many of us don't have the willpower to Exercise, so we need activities with a purpose besides getting fit.

Think about how you can recreate one or two of the older ways that made us more active – things that would work in your own life. You have to make a real need, not a pretend one. For example, saying you will walk up the stairs at work rather than take the lift won't work because the lift is still there waiting to be used.

But if you decide to save money by using a train station one stop nearer work – which means you have a fifteen minutes' walk to the station rather than three minutes – then you create a natural and real need to walk an extra twenty-four minutes a day. Leave with only just enough time to spare to catch the train both ways and you create a natural and real need to hurry – thus improving cardiovascular fitness as well as burning calories.

- Is there room in your life for a dog? I have several dog-owning friends, none of whom is overweight and all of whom are fit. The dog creates the absolute need to go out and walk twice a day, every day. Or you can buy a dog-jogging attachment – the springer – for your bike.
- Would you consider giving up your car? Taking taxis when you really can't use public transport works out much cheaper for town dwellers than running a car, in my experience. The rest of the time, it is often quicker to walk to where you are going than to get caught in traffic jams or wait for buses or trains. It is certainly quicker to cycle. Walking and cycling are two of the very best ways to get and stay fit and slim.
- Consider creating a vegetable garden and work several hours a week in it to grow your own veg. You'll save money while you get fitter. Or you might, like my neighbour the author, John Lewis Stempel, go one better and try living off the land for a year – he not only lost weight and got very fit but saved a fortune too. (More about John and his philosophy in the next chapter.)
- If you are the kind of person who enjoys competing and enjoys winning then think about any competitive sport (except darts, of course), and give it a go. Research shows you're much more likely to continue to be active if your activity involves other people and not letting them down.

And as for your kids, don't ignore the gnawings of guilt when you see them in front of a screen yet again. Take them to the park or for a nature or sightseeing walk, or play sport with them at the local leisure centre – shared activity is an even better family cement and pleasure than eating together.

It takes determination to undo not only your ingrained habits, but also the changes that mankind has forced upon itself over many years. But interestingly, our world may be forcing us to do exactly that, as global warming may cause a new need for us to rethink our couch potato power-driven habits. As fuel prices soar and fuel itself runs out, long daily commutes by car or train may no longer be normal or even possible. In the long term, we may need to think about the environment, as well as our purses, and return to a way of life where we use our own manpower more and live a more natural – and active – life.

In the short term, however, the ideas I've given above are just some of the ways in which you might create a need to be active that works for you.

✶ *The health connection*

Lastly, but by no means least, there is the need, which has to be mentioned, to be healthy if you want to live a full and varied life. If you're young, slim and in good health, you are probably unlikely to peer into the future and worry about things like arthritis, heart attacks, diabetes or clogged arteries or whether you'll die aged sixty or ninety. Health protection is a bit like taking out a pension – not something many people under thirty ever consider. The health need may resonate more with older people, but it is there, none the less, for everyone.

So let's look at some of the benefits activity can bring us in terms of our health:

- Two long-term large studies of people from middle age onwards have found that being fit is more important than being slim as we age – those who don't exercise suffer sharper physical decline.
- Cardiovascular fitness reduces the risks of heart disease and stroke by around 50 per cent and cancer by a third.

In addition, it's been shown that exercise can:

- improve depression by around 50 per cent; for some people with depression, physical activity can be as effective as counselling or medication
- improve memory and mental agility
- burn calories and, in some circumstances, body fat, thus helping weight control
- protect bones from osteoporosis
- help protect against joint and muscular stiffness and tension
- help you to relax and relieve mental and physical stress and tension, depending on the type of activity you do
- possibly improve your sex life, regulate hormones and minimise period pains
- help you to sleep
- improve eyesight

DIET OR EXERCISE?
A programme conducted by two UK universities, which encouraged women not to diet, but to take part in exercise classes found significant improvements in health and mental wellbeing. After a year, the women had lost some weight and were much fitter and happier with themselves. Women who took part in the scheme lost an average of 3.2kg (7lb) during the first three months, whereas women in the control group put on the same amount on average.

✱ *The fitness–food–health connection*
A flow chart

Small, regular increase in your activity level
↓
Small improvements in your well-being and feelings of self-esteem
↓
More incentive to eat well and look after your body
↓
Small improvements in your weight and shape
↓
More incentive to take regular activity
↓
More and ongoing improvements in your well-being,
fitness, health, size and shape
↓
Continuing long-term incentive to eat well and look after your body.

Want

I've found that a high proportion of women actually dislike or even fear exercise. I conducted an unscientific but interesting poll among friends and colleagues which highlighted the following negative feelings around exercise:

- It's exhausting.
- It hurts.
- It creates the feeling of being about to have a heart attack – it's dangerous!
- It makes you sweat.

- It's reminiscent of hated schooldays and it's humiliating; brings back memories of always being the last one to be chosen for the rounders team.
- It's boring and takes too long.
- It doesn't fit into a busy life.
- It creates hunger.
- It's pointless.

And something a lot of women feel:

- I'm just no good at it; I like doing things I'm good at.

✱ *The primary want*

While people will put up with the most rigorous diets because they desperately *want* the end (short-term) result – i.e. to be slimmer – this doesn't work so well for exercise because people aren't so bothered about being fit. Madonna arms? Don't need them. A washboard tummy? Don't care – just wear a one-piece on the beach. You can't really see fitness, that's why. You don't walk down the street in summer and think people are talking about you behind your back because you don't have a six-pack. But you may just feel that way if you're fat.

As you're reading this book though, chances are that you *do* have concerns about your weight, that you do *want* to escape from the fat trap for life and that you *want* to have a body you feel good inside. Well – exercise can not only help you lose weight or reshape, it is also *the best* way there is of keeping the weight off for good. And that must surely be the ultimate, 'the primary' want?

The stark, simple truth is that if you're sedentary you'll find it harder to lose weight and much harder to keep it off; if you're active, you'll find it easier to lose weight and much easier to keep it off. Research proves this.

✱ *Creating the want*

Having already created the need (see pp. 166–8), you have given exercise a more discernible purpose – which should, in itself, make it much more likely that you will want it. So next, you have to find ways to banish the negatives/obstacles and make the positives so enticing and enjoyable that you've just *got* to do it.

To this end, I've enlisted the help of my friend and colleague Lizzie Webb, the TV exercise guru. Lizzie has spent much of her adult life changing people's attitudes to exercise and making it more enjoyable and do-able.

- **Exercise is exhausting/hurts/is dangerous.**
  If exercise is all these things, you are doing something wrong. Simple as that. We've already touched on listening to your body to discover your own fitness IQ – the line between not enough and too much? Well, this is a good place to talk about body IQ in a bit more detail.

  If, up until now, you have been a couch potato and you start exercising like a mad thing, you are likely to feel exhausted or hurt very quickly. You may wake up the next day, aching all over, and decide to call it a day, as far as exercise is concerned.

  It's important to understand that the level, duration and difficulty of any activity you begin needs to be in inverse proportion to your fitness, so the more unfit you are, the less you should do. This is particularly true if you are obese, as vigorous exercise can stress the joints.

  So be sensible: start small, do it regularly, build up gradually and keep it up!

DID YOU KNOW?
Research shows that not only can caffeine help improve stamina while exercising, it can also diminish muscular pain experienced during exercise. One strong cup of coffee before a workout may be enough to make a real difference.

- **Exercise makes you sweat.**
  Says Lizzie: 'What is wrong with sweating? Working up a little sweat through exercise is one of the first signs that it's working – so don't knock it. You will sweat if you're raising your heart rate and benefiting your heart, and its purpose is to help prevent you from overheating. You exercise in a comfy old top and trackies, do your activity and have a shower. No need to worry about how you look.' Sweating also provides a much better 'detox' than many that you'd actually pay for. Another reason not to knock it.

- **It's reminiscent of hateful schooldays and it's humiliating …**
  The memories of being the unchosen one or of being humiliated by the sports teacher in front of all the others because you kept dropping the ball or couldn't climb the rope can be hard to shake off. Says Lizzie: 'Pick something that doesn't remind you of school

and which you can do without feeling inadequate. Dancing is exercise – most people love dancing and if you pick the right sort, you can do it any way you like without anyone being able to tell you you're not doing it well enough or doing it all wrong.'

For people with deep-seated trauma about PE in their schooldays and exercise in general, I suggest avoiding all competitive and team sports at least to begin with, and choosing activities where no one, least of all yourself, is judging you or even looking at you. The Wii in the sitting room might be a fun idea to get you started or even simply dancing to a fitness DVD. Or for companionship without edge, a rambling club is a good idea. Once you are fitter and more confident you might take the plunge.

- **It's boring and takes too long.**
  As we've seen, exercise is not just one thing, it can be any of a number of things, so lumping it all together as one 'boring' activity is illogical. What's boring for one person (treadmill anyone?) may well be enjoyable for the next. (Although I defy anyone to find, say, a cycle ride with the wind in their hair and great views boring … that's soul food, not exercise.)
  As for taking too long, if that's the case, you're either doing the wrong thing or doing it for too long. When you start out, unfit, you do need patience because – as explained above – you need to start small and gradually increase.
  So, if you're easily bored, here are four happy facts:
  1. You can do your cardio activity in three ten-minute bursts a day, according to DoH and USA guidelines – so, ten minutes skipping, ten cycling and ten rowing, for example.
  2. As a rule of thumb, one minute of vigorous-intensity activity is about the same as two minutes' moderate-intensity activity in helping you to get fit and burn calories. If you can get fit enough to work at an intense level, you get all the benefits in half the time.
  3. There is a lot you can do while doing something else that bores you less: you can peddle on a mini-bike under your desk while you work or play on the computer; you can listen to music while you walk or run or do gym work (there are music tracks specifically designed to complement the pace of your workout – see Further Help, p. 218 – and research shows that people exercise harder and keep going for longer if they listen to music); you can stretch on the floor while you watch TV; there is even fitness equipment (e.g. Gamercize) that

works with your games console – so if you stop pedalling or stepping, your game stops too.

4. The Green Gym (see Further Help, p. 221) is a great way to work out and do something interesting at the same time, and in this case help to conserve the countryside in the process. You could also try eco-running (or walking). It's the latest idea from the USA – you take a litter sack with you, go out for your run or walk and pick up whatever litter you see on the way (but do wear gloves!).

Finally I'd like to mention the rugby player Jonny Wilkinson, whose dedication to training is legendary. He keeps going, he says, by concentrating on the immediate task, the next ten yards, even the next step, but never the whole task.

- **Exercise doesn't fit into a busy life.**
  This is something I hear a lot, in particular from mums with preschool – age children, especially under one year old. They can't figure out how to fit in exercise with a child in tow (see Further Help, pp. 220–1). In fact, pushing a buggy is itself quite good exercise; and many sports centres now have their own crèche. For mobile kids there's plenty you can do outdoors with them, as well as swimming and family activities at the leisure centre. For people with busy careers the best way to look at it is that you may be able to work faster and/or more efficiently if your brain and body are oxygenated through exercise. And you will definitely benefit from the regular 'me' time. (See also '… it takes too long', above.)

- **Exercise creates hunger.**
  Studies into the effects of exercise on hunger have produced varying results. One conducted in America in 2005 found that high-intensity workouts were followed by food intake that replaced 90 per cent of the calories burnt, while lower-intensity workouts resulted in only a third of the energy being replaced. In the UK, Dr David Stensel, a sports scientist, has more recently found an interesting paradox – that if you are cold when you exercise (e.g. in a cool swimming pool) you crave high-fat foods afterwards, whereas 'hot' exercise, e.g. walking on a hot day, dulls the appetite – probably because heat suppresses the appetite-stimulating hormone, ghrelin. Stensel also found that moderate walking didn't increase hunger at all, whatever the temperature. Lastly, short periods of exercise are more likely to increase appetite, while long bouts of activity produce appetite suppression.

And finally, there is a psychological element to post-exercise hunger, too – if they've been 'good' and exercised, some people use food as a reward.

So my advice is that for people who crave chocolate or chips straight after a workout, it's best to exercise in heat, rather than cold (happily, warm muscles are less likely to get strained) and to do moderate to long-length exercise rather than short, sharp bursts.

- **Exercise is pointless.**
  It's clear from the list of benefits on p. 168 that activity isn't pointless from a health perspective, and the ways in which you can use your body instead of resources, such as petrol, to go places and get things done shows it can and should have purpose in your everyday life. But lastly, exercise can also help you get and keep a slimmer and more efficient body.

GOALS AND TARGETS

Keeping a diary and setting targets are simple motivational tools that really do work; they're why people return to computer games and puzzles day after day – because they want to improve their scores/results/times etc. It's also been found that women are more inclined to continue with exercise, as well as with diet, if they tell people about their plans, get encouragement from friends and family and have particular goals in mind – getting fit for a charity run, for example.

Need and want - conclusion

Going back to the idea of that 'primary want', remember that exercise:

- helps burn calories, so you can either lose weight slightly quicker or eat a little more
- helps raise your metabolic rate – and one of the best ways is to strengthen your muscles and increase their size, as your metabolic rate increases as your muscle tissue does
- promotes tighter, toned muscles which help improve your shape and posture

In the next chapter, there are tools to help you create your own need and want, including self-discovery questionnaires and outcome suggestions. But for now, let's give Lizzie the last word here:

> 'Your motivation? I always say that you have one body and it is down to you to take care of it. You have control over it! And in this life, it is often the one thing that you have control over. Controlling your body should be a pleasure, not a punishment – so turn it into a positive. There is little quite as good as the feeling you get from having a body that works for you, a body you can enjoy. Looks aren't so important, but if your body functions as well as it can – which it will through exercise – then you can feel proud.'

Exercise – Where to Find What You Need

You may have noticed that although there is an exercise chapter in the book, there are no formal recommendations – no set of exercises, no specific programmes for you to follow for aerobic workouts, strength or flexibility. The reason for this is that I know you can take very good DVDs out of the library or go online and find all the information you need to get started within minutes. (Plus, the Further Help section at the back of this book gives you some good starting points too.) So I've chosen not to focus on all this here.

However, you do need some knowledge in order to achieve what you want with your activities, so here are some broad guidelines which may help you.

Don't be taken in

As with the slimming aids, diets and foods we looked at earlier in the book, the fitness industry is awash with gimmicky (and often very expensive) 'exercise aids' and people who are trying to make a living out of your unfit body. There no quick fixes for getting fit or for losing weight via exercise. Any weight you lose through normal amounts of exercise – i.e. a few hours a week – will be in the region of 0.2kg (half a pound) or so a week, or less.

If you are carrying an excess of body fat, you can't 'spot-reduce' parts of your body, such as your stomach, by exercise. You can firm up the muscles under the flab, but you can't spot reduce the flab in any particular area. If you want a flat washboard stomach, you need to reduce your overall body fat. So be sure to avoid any equipment (or teacher) promising that you can spot-reduce.

Also, be very wary of any exercise equipment or aid that promises shaping up and/or weight loss without effort. If it feels too easy, then it probably isn't working. So it isn't aerobic if you aren't breathing harder, it isn't toning you up if you don't have to work your muscles and it isn't stretching you if you can't feel a stretch. If you are unsure about a fitness method, class or trainer, check out the industry's own self-regulatory body, the Fitness Industry Association (see Further Help p. 220).

A MYTH ABOUT FAT BURNING

There's a lot of nonsense talked about 'fat burning' when you exercise. The myth goes that you need to do exercise which burns body fat itself for fuel, rather than using your carb/glycogen stores.

But if you burn up your carb/glycogen stores, you're still using calories from your body's 'calorie pool', that can't be later converted into fat.

What matters for weight control is doing enough exercise to create a calorie deficit over time.

Don't spend too much of your hard-earned cash

It is very easy to spend a lot of money in the quest to get fit. But I can't find any research that shows that the more you spend, the more successful you'll be at getting and staying fit. Indeed, many people who lash out the cash for an expensive gym membership in a sudden burst of enthusiasm don't attend often enough to make the outlay worthwhile, especially if the gym is not close to either home or work. A local council-run facility, which is generally a lot less expensive, may be a good compromise.

✱ The gym

In theory, a gym might not be a bad idea. A good one should have equipment for increasing your strength/muscle mass and for your aerobic quotient, and is especially useful during dark winter evenings or rainy days, when outdoor activity is not so enticing. But the fact is that many people just don't like the gym. Womens'-only gyms (see Further Help p. 220) may be preferable for some.

If you have some space you can set aside at home for your own gym equipment, this can end up cheaper than a gym membership and it will save you time too. However, be careful when choosing equipment, as some cheap-end machines will disappoint and bore you after a few weeks because, like an underpowered car, they can't offer higher levels of workout intensity. If you do choose the home gym option, go for a (free) induction at the gym first, so you know how to use your equipment properly. It's also well worth buying some of the lower-cost pieces of equipment too – a set of weights, a dumbbell, some resistance bands, a gymball, a mini trampoline are all good, honest pieces.

✱ Personal trainers

At about £50 an hour, personal trainers are even more expensive than a club membership. But yes, they are motivating, and may be able to tell and show you a great deal about your own body and how to keep it running well.

EXERCISE INTENSITY LEVELS

The intensity of cardiovascular (aerobic, stamina-building) exercise can be described as strenuous or moderate. Mild activity is that which achieves little aerobic benefit at all. But what constitutes a strenuous, moderate or mild activity for you will depend on your current fitness level. For example, for an elite long-distance track athlete, running 1.6km (1 mile) in ten minutes would count as moderate or even mild, whereas for most other people, it would be strenuous (and for many, even unwise, dangerous or just not possible).

As a guide, moderate-intensity exercise will make you warm, slightly out of breath, and maybe sweat a little. If you're feeling very hot and very out of breath, it is no longer moderate.

Examples

- **Mild:** light daily activities, such as shopping, cooking or doing the laundry don't count towards the guidelines for aerobic (cardiovascular) fitness because your body isn't working hard enough to get your heart rate up. These activities do all 'count', however, in other ways: they all burn up more calories than just sitting in a chair (e.g. standing at the cooker uses around two calories a minute, while sitting uses around one), and thus can help you stay a reasonable weight, and they may have strength or flexibility benefits too (stretching to hang clothes on a washing line, for example, or bending to polish a low shelf).
- **Moderate:** walking briskly, low-impact aerobics class, riding a bike on level ground, pushing a lawnmower, ballroom dancing.
- **Strenuous:** jogging or running, swimming laps, cycling uphill, Latin dancing, squash.

Alternatively, you could go to a local class with a competent instructor and small numbers, where, especially if you ask, you may get practically the same help for a fraction of the price.

* Virtual trainers
Almost as good as a personal trainer may be a Wii Fit programme – especially if you already have a Nintendo console in the house. For £70 or so for the software you have a whole range of exercises designed personally for you and can do them any time, whatever the weather.)

* Books/DVDs
Of the two, a DVD is better than a book, as you can actually see the instructor moving. Books with photographs or line drawings can be open to misinterpretation; the models in exercise photos are often doing things wrongly or even dangerously, while an illustrator is working from photos, or sometimes even just stick people drawn for them by the author. (I've been there; I know!)

But don't forget: for every aspect of fitness, there is an activity which is free. As we saw on pp. 166–8, if you make more room for everyday 'lifestyle' activities, they could even be all that you need – and for many of us, these are the most pleasant ways to get fit of all.

Exercise Regimes and Activities – What They Will Really Do For You

Note: all calorie burns given here are just a guide; the heavier you are, the more you will burn.

Formal (gym or teacher-led) exercise

* Aerobics class
There are many types of class that will give you a cardio workout, including 'dance aerobics' (exercise to music at varying levels), jazzercise, kickboxing, step class (stepping up and down on a box). Most types will also have some toning effect on the lower body and abdominals, and some may have a slight flexibility benefit. Prices are reasonable, but most people only go once a week.
Calorie burn: 6–7 per minute

✱ Pilates

Not for cardio, but helps make the body stronger and more supple and can improve posture. There's a lot of balancing work, which beginners often find difficult. Ten Pilates is hardest of all. The UK's Chartered Society of Physiotherapy believes that up to three quarters of people who do Pilates-type exercises don't do them properly, which can cause back pain.
Calorie burn: 4 per minute

✱ Power plate

This piece of equipment costs from around £2000 up to £7000 (or you can find it in some gyms); it is said to provide a sixty-minute muscle workout (by vibrating up to fifty times a second) in just ten minutes. It's not as easy as you might think and there's no real cardio benefit, but a six-month Belgian study found that power plate users lost two thirds more organ fat (the dangerous kind that is stored around the body's organs) than people who were just cutting calories or doing aerobic exercise. The Wii Fit balance board and programme could achieve similar muscle-toning effects for less cost.
Calorie burn: 4 per minute

✱ Rowing machine

Great way to burn calories and exercise your arms, back and stomach. Beware of cheap, small machines that don't allow you full extension or improvement. If you can't afford a decent one, use one at a council leisure centre instead.
Calorie burn: 8 per minute

✱ Stepper/stairmaster

Like walking uphill, but harder, a stepper is one of the quickest ways to burn calories, but beginners should start on the very lowest resistance or on easier equipment. Excellent thigh and butt toner and also works abdomen. A cheaper option would be to climb stairs, although you do waste time because you have to come back down to keep climbing, which is why you only burn around 6 calories a minute.
Calorie burn: 9 per minute

> **FACT**
> In New York, running up stairs is a recognised sport. The winner of the last run up the Empire State Building's eighty-six floors did it in just over ten minutes.

✳ Spinning

No, sitting and making cotton won't get you slim, but spinning here is a fancy name for an indoor static cycling class and, as with any exercise bike, if you pedal hard enough you'll burn masses of calories and get very fit. Great for toning thighs and calves too.

Calorie burn: 6–7 per minute

✳ Weight training

While weight training isn't an aerobic activity as such, it does burn quite a lot of calories, as the effort required is big; it also builds muscle over time, which helps speed your metabolic rate – your MR is raised for several hours after training, and higher weights/fewer repeats produces better results than lower weights/more repeats.

In one study, participants in a three-month strength-training programme gained 1.4kg (3lb) of muscle and lost 1.8kg (4lb) of fat, on average, while eating 15 per cent more calories each day.

A set of free weights/dumbbells can achieve results as good as using the fixed weights at the gym, but if you do go that route, get a good weight-training DVD or other programme to follow. Resistance bands – cheap to buy – are quite good for taking with you when travelling, and using your own body weight as resistance (e.g. press-ups) is quite good too, but neither is as effective as proper weight training.

Calorie burn: 4–5 per minute

✳ Yoga

Similar results to Pilates, creating a longer, leaner look and making you more supple with some resistance involved. Mostly not for cardio, but ashtanga yoga involves much more movement and can be aerobic. Yoga can also reduce stress-related eating. A New Zealand study found that women who did yoga and meditation to relax, but didn't follow any particular diet plan, lost weight and kept it off. Some yoga poses are not good for bad backs, though others can actually help. Beginners may find completing some of the poses hard – choose a class to suit your level.

Calorie burn: 4 per minute or 6–7 for ashtanga

Informal exercise

✱ *Cycling*
Excellent aerobic exercise and great for thigh and calf strength; also helps abdominals, but has no impact on upper body or flexibility (in fact, it can make flexibility worse, if done for long periods and depending on the style of bike).
Calorie burn: 5–8 per minute, depending on terrain

✱ *Dancing*
All medium- and fast-paced dancing has some aerobic benefit – the quicker the pace, the more of a cardio workout you're getting, based on how much of the time your feet are off the floor. Again, depending on dance type, you'll also get a reasonable flexibility workout – but only break-dancing will improve strength. Most of us may be better off lifting a few weights, rather than trying street moves.
Calorie burn: 4–9 per minute, depending on type

✱ *Gardening*
Heavy gardening, such as digging or shovelling manure, can provide aerobic, strength and some flexibility benefits. Mowing can be a good or very good cardio workout, depending on the type of mower used (ride-ons don't count!).
Calorie burn: 4–6 per minute

✱ *Horse riding*
Well yes, the horse does do most of the work, but if you proceed at a steady trot, you'll be burning calories too, as well as tightening your butt, thighs and abdomen. Non-dressage riding, though, does little for flexibility and nothing for upper-body strength (unless you have a puller, of course).
Calorie burn: 5–6 per minute at a trot

✱ *Housework*
One survey suggested that women spend up to sixteen hours a week doing housework, to which I say – not in this house they don't. The trouble with 'housework' is that it could include anything from cleaning the washbasin with an antiseptic wipe (no calories burnt) to polishing a 30-ft entrance hall by hand (many calories burnt). On average, we probably spend most time vacuum cleaning, dusting and doing laundry, but even these can be fairly non-strenuous tasks. Unless you have to fling open the windows and strip off your jumper while you're doing house chores (that means you're hot, which means you're burning calories), it's unlikely to be aerobic. You may need a bit of strength to lift the laundry, and a bit of flexibility to hang washing or bend to

clean a nook or cranny. But housework as reliable exercise for overall fitness is a bit of a tricky one. (That said, of course, every little helps – and the more you put into each task, physically, the better it is. And don't forget to run up and down the stairs too, as you work, if you have any.)

Calorie burn: 2–5 per minute, depending on chore

✳ Ice skating/skating

Because the blades or wheels reduce friction, the amount of energy you expend will be less than in some other 'travelling' forms of exercise, such as jogging or brisk walking. However these are still useful forms of activity, not least because they're so enjoyable; and inline-skating can be a useful type of transport in urban areas.

Few or no flexibility/strength benefits.

Calorie burn: 4–5 per minute

✳ Jogging/running

I want to weep when I see people slow-jogging along the pavements, red in the face, pained expression, technically jogging, but actually going at no more than walking pace – and, almost always, looking unfit and unhappy. Most people would be better off brisk walking than trying to jog or run on hard surfaces. Yes, for fit people with good footwear, running is a great way to burn calories and stay fit, but even then, the impact may be a problem. (Research shows that many regular runners will face joint problems later in life.) With an eye on my joints, I'd rather cycle or swim, and would much rather walk, even if I have to spend a bit longer doing it.

Calorie burn: 8–14 per minute

MYTH – RUNNING BURNS MORE CALORIES

People often say that you'll burn more calories running a mile than walking a mile. However, that is not the case. In actual fact, you burn approximately 62 calories for every 45.3kg (100lb) of body weight for every 1.6km (1 mile) you cover on foot, regardless of whether you slow-walk, jog or run fast. If you run, however, you'll do the mile quicker, of course. So the statement should be: 'You'll burn more calories running for half an hour than you will walking for half an hour.'

✳ Skiing

Downhill skiing is a bit like ice skating – the gradient, the low resistance run and the skies do most of the work (but it's wonderful for thigh strength). Should you be in Norway any time, though, try cross-country (Nordic) skiing. It's a killer! You'll burn as many calories a minute as you would running or going full out on the rowing machine.

Gym skiing machines (elliptical trainers) have a similar calorie-burning effect, although they may not leave you feeling as exhausted as the real thing. *Calorie burn:* 9 per minute (cross country); 5–6 per minute (downhill)

✱ Skipping

Brilliant, cheap and simple aerobic exercise, which also helps balance and lower-body strength. One drawback is that it takes quite a while to be able to do continuous skipping for even ten minutes, as it's hard work. Not, therefore, for the beginner. Nor is it for anyone who lives in a restricted space. But great for a workout if you're quite fit and have a park across the road or a garden. *Calorie burn:* 7 per minute

✱ Swimming

Swimming works every muscle in your body and is low impact as the water carries your weight – this means it can be a good choice for anyone with conditions such as arthritis or joint pain. It's also inexpensive, if you have access to a council-run pool. It is time-consuming though, taking into account travel, changing, showering and a forty-five-minute swim. Aqua aerobics classes can be a good option if you find lengths boring – you'll tone up a bit, but you won't burn many calories. *Calorie burn for swimming lengths:* 6–9 per minute

✱ Walking

If you do it briskly, walking is good aerobic exercise and tones up the lower body, but doesn't do a lot for the upper (except, if you walk up- or downhill, it will work your abs). Walking can either serve a purpose (e.g. walking to work) or it can be fun (say, if you join a rambling or orienteering club, walk to a good view or an old church). A simple pedometer, which counts your steps and times you, is also a cheap motivator – you could aim for 10,000 steps a day, for example. Wearing the pedometer all day long is a good way of seeing how much exercise you get during your normal activities. *Calorie burn:* 5–7 per minute

Competitive sports

According to Sport England, over 6 million English adults over sixteen play sport at least three times a week. But the truth is that for most of us out-of-condition, slightly overweight people, getting fit by taking part in competitive sports isn't really an option. You need to gain a degree of fitness using some of the options outlined above. Then, look at doing whatever it was you were best at when you were young, as a starting point. The various official sports bodies across the UK (see Further Help, p. 220) can give you information about particular sport facilities in your area. Another idea is to start an activity that can become a 'sport' if you want it to, later, such as cycling or swimming.

A word of warning about participating in 'team sports': a lot of them involve quite a bit of 'hanging around', rather than being active, depending on the sport and the position in which you play. There's also a danger of injury with many sports. Even so, most will help you stay fit and healthy and they come with a strong motivation factor – other people around you, wanting you to do well. They can also be great fun – why not try Ultimate Frisbee, for example, or extreme pogo?

In conclusion then, as to the question of your own fitness quotient it is the amount of activity you take which fits the following five criteria:

1. You don't find it daunting, you can fit it into your life and will stick with it.
2. It's not so easy that you feel as if you're not doing anything.
3. You feel – and maybe look – better than you did (these benefits will mostly take a while to show themselves, though even after one session you will probably feel more mentally sharp and happier with yourself).
4. You are using the current official guidelines as a blueprint, even if you don't do quite as much, or do a bit more.
5. You do what feels right for you – if it feels too hard, it probably is too hard; if it feels too easy, it's too easy; and if it makes you unhappy, you should swap to something different. As Lizzie says, you are in control and you should exercise not only your body, but also your integrity and your common sense.

And remember: *any* activity at all is better than none. If you can't do 'enough' – do some!

10

All In The Mind

What's Keeping You from Taking Control?

Up to now, this book has been about examining the strange and often conflicting worlds of size, shape, body image, food intake and exercise levels and about trying to make some sense of it all. By now, you'll realise that your food and activity behaviours are often governed by outside influences, as well as by habit, convenience and want. You will also have laid all the myths to rest and formed a clear picture of what you might achieve with your body, size, shape and health, why it might be a good idea and how to go about it. In other words, you've got your body IQ.

In order to escape the fat trap for good though, what you need to know now is what's stopping you.

Goals, Incentives, Rewards and Punishments – Do They Work?

Since the beginning of human society people have been bullied – or bullied themselves – into doing things they don't really want to do with the incentive of reward or the threat of punishment. And when it comes to weight loss or maintenance, it's no different.

Slimming clubs use all of these strategies to motivate people and keep them on track. The weekly weigh-in and/or the target weight loss are goals, but also potential punishments, in that if you don't meet the targets, you lose face. There are even online betting sites where people pledge their own money against losing weight by a set time. And some people may be motivated by the partner who threatens to leave them if they don't lose weight or the suspicion that they were passed over for the job of their dreams because they're obese.

There are also positive motivational tools. You might promise yourself a holiday, a party or a new car if you lose the weight. Or you might raise money for a local charity by getting sponsorship for every kilogram you lose. Or you might have a particular event in mind – your wedding, your fortieth birthday – for which you want to get in shape.

There is no doubt that such ideas – carrot or stick; take your pick – do work for some people (and some more than others), but in my experience, while they may provide fantastic short-term motivation, they rarely achieve long-term success. Once the motivational tool or support mechanism is taken away, there is nothing to stop you falling back – and that's yo-yo dieting by another name. Which is why most slimming clubs encourage their successful members to return to the group regularly (often with free membership) so that they keep motivated.

What most of us need, perhaps, is the long-term desire – or willpower – to change, coupled with small, occasional incentives along the way. Incentives without the long-term desire are unlikely to work. And I believe that the desire to change – in this instance, to eat a more natural diet – will come once you truly believe that you will enjoy it.

Finding the Will

Perhaps the first thing you should do is to go back and read Chapter Two again. If you're struggling with lack of willpower, lack of incentive, inability to resist the temptation of chocolate or cream cakes, Chapter Two will remind you of how we weren't built that way – how we have all been programmed by external forces to think we enjoy eating these things. Next, decide whether you want to be your own person or controlled by people who do not have your best interests at heart. I know which I prefer.

Here's a story, by way of illustration. Many years ago, after several failed attempts, I managed to give up smoking suddenly and very easily. I sat in my office, about to open a fresh packet of cigarettes, when I looked at it and experienced a moment of clarity. I felt annoyed with the packet, and the fact that I was sitting there holding it. I asked myself: 'Do I want to be controlled by an inanimate object?' The answer was a resounding 'No'. I suddenly got very angry – angry with the cigarette company for enslaving me for years; angry with the packet; angry with myself, for being controlled by something so insignificant and so negative. In that moment, I found whatever it took to throw the packet away and have never bought one since. I had found my motivation. Neither the health risk nor the wasted money had been enough to do it. But my anger was enough.

It is only once you believe that your actions should be controlled by you and not by others, that you will find the motivation to make the changes that will benefit you. And finding your own personal motivation – that thing that really spurs you on, regardless of whatever anyone/thing else is telling you – is central to your overall success.

First though, you need the confidence to believe you *can* do it.

Mindful Eating

Taking control means taking responsibility for yourself and your actions. You can train your brain to take control with the application of 'mindful eating'. The term 'mindful eating' was coined to refer to eating in a greener, more environmentally conscious way, but can also be applied to what we put in our mouths in more general, health-giving terms.

Hunger/appetite, greed, addiction: why we've lost the plot around food ... and what to do about it

Mindful eating can help us to differentiate between hunger, greed and appetite – and, indeed, satiety. As we've seen, the bullying tactics of the modern food industry have stripped us of the tools we need to tell the difference, so we eat because we can, not because we need or even want to.

We can also use mindful eating to help us overcome eating for emotional reasons. While food should be enjoyable, and can also be life-enhancing, relaxing and exciting, it should not be used as a prop. Eating for emotional reasons (when you're upset, angry, bored, depressed, lonely and so on) does not cancel the emotion (for more than, perhaps, a very short while) and can increase negativity by introducing emotions such as guilt, misery or even self-loathing into the equation. It also eventually overrides your natural ability to recognise true hunger.

✱ Hunger/appetite?
How long is it since you felt real hunger pangs? Can you tell whether what you are experiencing is real hunger? Here are some pointers:

Real hunger/true appetite
- You are feeling hunger pangs in your stomach.
- Your stomach is rumbling.
- It is quite a long time since you last ate anything.

Fake hunger/false appetite
- You've caught the aroma of baking and it makes you feel peckish.

- You're bored, so food comes into your head.
- You've seen someone else eating.
- You've just eaten your fill, but a splendid dessert is put in front of you; suddenly you feel hungry again.

Try setting yourself a hunger scale from one to ten – where ten is very hungry and one is not at all hungry – and only eat if you can truly say you are over eight. A friend of mine does this and it works very well.

✱ *Greed?*

Greed (when applied to food) is the excessive desire to eat more than you need, according to the dictionary. But I think that is a massive simplification. If you eat when you're not hungry, you are not necessarily greedy. Research shows that obese people don't have the same 'I am full' mechanism as slimmer people, so someone you might describe as greedy may, in fact, have a physiological problem.

And most of us don't overeat for greed, but for emotional reasons or simply out of habit. We've forgotten how to say, 'No thanks, I'm not hungry', or 'That's it, I've had enough'. We have to remind ourselves that we can find food to eat if we really do feel hungry later. We're not going to starve.

RELEARNING FOOD PREFERENCES

You might find it hard to believe, but there is plenty of evidence to show that relearning preferences is a much easier business than you would imagine. If you want to do it.

Two years ago, John Lewis Stempel, the farmer and author of *The Wild Life* whom I mentioned in Chapter Nine, was slightly overweight and had a weakness for starchy foods. Then, he got the idea to try to live off the land around his home in Herefordshire for a year and write a diary of how he got on. He stuck it out and a year after the end of his experiment, he feels his eating habits have changed for good:

'At first, I had cravings for starchy, bun-like things – I was fixated with McDonald's burger baps, and had visions of Bath Olivers night and day.

It was like a detoxing programme. For the first three to four days I had a headache, hunger pangs – so bad it was real pain – nausea and felt weak, but that didn't last long. Then I became very clear-headed. I believe hunter-gatherers had little food but their brains adapted – they had to remain clear-headed to survive.

I lost a stone in a week. The cravings had mostly gone after a month. I also lost my sweet tooth, although I still ate honey and hedgerow fruits. Over the course of the year, I changed shape and got more muscle from being active, hunting and walking.

As I was losing my taste for starchy and refined foods, I found my palate becoming much sharper – I was able to detect and enjoy a whole range of new tastes. I think in primitive times humans would have been able to select to help maintain health and heal – I notice that when farm animals are off colour and allowed free grazing, they pick the leaves that will help them recover.'

A year on, John feels his experiment has taught him things about the relationship with food that will stay with him for life:

'I don't eat refined foods in the way I used to. My feeling on refined starches is that they don't exist in nature, so they have no real purpose in a more natural life. At the end of the year, when I tried refined sweet foods again, I was nauseated. Although at last I could return to eating what I wanted, taking my pick from the supermarket – I didn't want to, and I couldn't. My stomach just couldn't take it.

And don't be afraid of hunger pangs – they are there to tell us when to eat. Lastly, I value food more now. I'm not fixated; I am relaxed about what I eat, but this helps me make judicious choices.'

I'm not suggesting you make changes as drastic as John did – simply that as much as you may not credit it, your palate can change, faster than you would think. If you keep in touch with what your body is saying and eat naturally, it will happen. This is backed up by research at Roehampton University, which has found that after a trigger food is given up, cravings cease. And, as Dr David Kessler, ex-head of the USA Food and Drug Administration, points out in his excellent book on why we overeat (see Further Help, p. 221), meat-lovers who turn vegetarian soon begin to view animal flesh as disgusting.

We've learnt to think of pap foods as rewards and treats and instead you need to think of items such as a piece of fresh fruit, a delicious vegetable soup or a plate of seafood as the true reward or treat – or offer yourself rewards/treats that are not food based at all.

✳ *Addiction?*

Are food addictions and cravings harder to beat than 'normal' overeating? Indeed, is there such a thing as true food addiction?

Dr Robert Hill, a leading specialist in addictions (see Further Help, p. 219), believes that the answer is both 'Yes' and 'No', depending on what one means by addiction. There is no evidence for physical *tolerance* and subsequent *withdrawal* states (the essence of addiction) in relation to food. However, viewed on another level, namely *dependence*, everyone is clearly addicted to food.

> 'The majority of people who have not eaten will experience cravings for food. Cravings can be thought of as a spur to action to seek out something that we want or need. In the case of food it can fulfil both a want and a need. Thus, we will all crave food when malnourished or starving, but why do we crave when we have sufficient calories?
>
> Part of the explanation lies in the behavioural associations that we have learnt to make between food and feeling good, suggesting that food fulfils a secondary psychological function. It is also thought likely that certain foods are more likely to result in a pleasurable response by activating certain neurotransmitters e.g. sugar increasing dopamine activity. Thus, some individuals will have a high level of food-related thoughts in the absence of any calorie requirement deficits. One can infer that this is related to the pleasure-like qualities of food, rather than any functional necessity.'

Hill says that we use food as a tool in many ways:

> 'Food can become a primary focus for a whole range of life difficulties and, at the serious end of the spectrum, psychological and psychiatric difficulties. For instance, bulimia and anorexia – although food-focused – are likely to be caused by non-food-related issues, e.g. control, perfectionism, self-punishment, thus food is merely a vehicle for trying to attain other ends.
>
> For the majority of people, periodic over-consumption of food will be related to anxiety and stress and occurs as a form of positive reward and/or as a means of controlling some part of their life when the rest of it feels out of control. This is a form of *negative reinforcement*, where food is used in order not to experience something unpleasant, i.e. the emotion of anxiety. The opposite, *positive reinforcement*, is when we do something for its rewarding properties in

and of itself. Thus the gourmet will eat for the sheer pleasure of food. A stressed gourmet on the other hand may eat simply to avoid feeling stressed (negative reinforcement), although they would probably still like their food (positive reinforcement).

People who overeat all the time may be conditioned by either positive or negative reinforcing factors. Understanding which is which is key to changing one's relationship to food.'

THE FOUR CYCLES OF CHANGE
The cycles or stages of change are often talked about in addiction. This model suggests that people go through four phases:
- Pre-contemplation – the addict doesn't think there is a problem
- Contemplation – maybe there is a problem; time to weigh up the pros and cons of change
- Action
- Maintenance or relapse

Knowing where you are in the cycle is important in determining what you should be doing. For example, if you are still in contemplation, an action plan will be premature and likely to fail, says Dr Hill.

Dr Hill's tips for beating food addiction
- Do something. There is evidence that a short period of activity (ten to fifteen minutes) can disrupt cravings. This is particularly helpful for boredom, which is often associated with snacking.
- Recognise that you may be ambivalent in your desire to change; if you weren't, change would be both easy and sustainable. Try doing a pros and cons exercise – the pros and cons of changing/not changing your eating habits.
- Have a reasonable and achievable goal that is broken down into mini-goals with clear behavioural steps concerning what you are going to do.
- Try to focus on what you are going to do, rather than what you are *not* going to do. Not doing something is far more difficult and, in many senses, burdensome than finding an alternative positive action.
- Understand the rule violation effect (RVE). There is a lot of evidence that when people have a fixed rule and then break it, they tend to give up and say things like 'in for a penny in for a pound'. Thus,

I may decide not to eat another chocolate in my life (probably not a reasonable or particularly achievable goal!). I then eat one and think, 'What the heck,' and eat the whole box. But a lapse does not have to turn into a relapse.

- Get to know your seemingly irrelevant decisions (SIDs). These are things that appear entirely reasonable on the surface, but are really a way of setting yourself up. An example would be popping into the petrol station (where they happen to serve your favourite pastries) to buy a paper!
- Be aware of all of your high-risk situations – those that are more likely to make you do the very thing you don't want to do. This could be an actual place or it could be an emotion. An example could be going to a buffet alone. This is probably a mixture of high-risk situation (plentiful grazing food) and emotion (I feel like a lemon, standing here on my own).
- Ask yourself whether food acts as a positive or negative reinforcer and try to understand its function in your life. The sensory impacts of supermarkets and restaurants are designed to maximise sales, therefore try and decide what you are going to eat or buy prior to entering these environments.

THE PROBLEM OF IMMEDIATE GRATIFICATION (PIG)

Dr Hill defines PIG as where a small immediate reward has a greater influence than a much larger, but delayed reward. He notes that food can be especially good at inducing the desire for immediate gratification, for example the smell of freshly baked cakes or roasted coffee. PIG is a particular problem in addiction to drugs and alcohol because of their immediate sensory effects and the very long delay between staying abstinent and feeling healthier. He argues that the same could be said of food.

But Professors Walter Mischel and Janet Metcalfe of Columbia University, USA, who elaborate on the PIG problem in their paper on willpower, say that it is possible to improve your control over the 'cold' area of the brain (the part that realises the fresh bread will be just a few moments in your mouth, while what is really important is your long-term goal to look better and feel more confident). They say that you can gently bully the hot area (the part that gets excited at the smell of the bread) into submission if you focus. And experiments prove that this becomes easier the more you practise.

- Carry a craving-busting card with you. This is a card with your top three tips for what you are going to do when you have a craving for food that you are trying to cut down or cut out. On the other side write down what it is you really want to achieve by changing your relationship to food.
- While it is important to understand your behaviour in relation to food, it is critical to become aware of your food-related thoughts and to understand and challenge these wherever possible. At the root of most unwanted behaviour is a permission-giving thought of some description.
- The responsibility to change is yours.

✷ Counselling

Cognitive behavioural therapy (CBT) is a popular form of therapy with a high success rate, and is especially good at helping people with addictions that almost always come with other integrated problems such as depression, stress or family issues. It can also help you come to terms with learnt behaviours around food – for example, you may have had it instilled in you as a child to finish everything on your plate, so that you've come to associate eating with obtaining approval.

CBT is available on the NHS and your doctor should be able to refer you if he or she agrees that it could be helpful. For people who can afford it, there are private CBT therapists nationwide (see Further Help, p. 221, for details).

Making Changes

To lose weight, you need to change your relationship with food. Unless you do that, it won't work long term. There are right and wrong ways of making changes. Here are the ways that work best:

- Make small changes for success. Large changes are often too daunting.
- Make only one new change at a time – whether it's giving up chocolate and giving up alcohol on the same day, or starting a healthy eating plan and moving house on the same day, more than one change in one go increases the chance of failure.
- Remember the rule of twenty-one – it takes up to twenty-one times to practise a new habit before it becomes a habit. If you can get to that figure it is 99 per cent likely that you will stick with it. So if you

decide to cut down your wine intake to one glass an evening, you may find it hard for twenty nights, but by the twenty-first night it will no longer be a problem. You will have created a new habit – and it will be easy.

- Forget about yesterday and tomorrow. Live in the present moment. This works well both for eating and activity strategies: no need to worry about yesterday's eating slip-ups or about all the future exercise sessions you plan to do. Concentrate on what you need to do now; nothing else really matters.

FIVE KEYS TO MINDFUL EATING

- Mindful eating begins in the shop (think about what you're buying) and continues in the kitchen (think about how you're preparing the food), then on throughout the meal.
- Stop and think before you eat: 'Do I really want it/need it?/Am I hungry?' If you aren't – try to spot the reason or reasons why you are considering eating anyway. Once you've spotted the reason, think of another way of dealing with it.
- It's harder to leave food on the plate than it is to finish a smaller plateful, so mindful eating begins in serving smaller portions.
- Eat slowly and concentrate on your food. As soon as you feel full, stop.
- Aim to feel good when you've finished eating. Before the meal, say the things you want to feel at the end of it: 'I want to feel good about myself. I want to feel energised. I want to feel satisfied, but not overfull.'

Stop Kidding Yourself

It's only when you stop fooling yourself as to why you're not changing your eating and lifestyle habits that you will really be able to do it.

I am often told, 'I can't afford to buy fresh fruit and vegetables,' or, 'How can I cook meals from scratch on what I earn?' But if you can splash out on cakes, biscuits, fizzy drinks, chocolate, pastries, takeaways, pizzas and so on, you can certainly afford a whole list of foods that are healthy and will help you maintain a good weight. Pulses of all sorts, wholegrains (including brown rice, bread and pasta), vegetables (e.g. cabbage) and fruit (e.g. apples during glut season) are all really cheap. And mackerel, herrings, eggs, many vegetables and fruits, some cheeses, milk, yogurt, chicken legs, liver are inexpensive too. Plus, a reduction in calorie intake and portion size will actually mean you can eat well for less, not more.

Another common excuse is, 'I'm way too busy to prepare healthy meals'. OK, it does take longer to make a meal from scratch than it does to heat a ready meal in the microwave. But with a little forward planning and the judicious purchase of healthy foods that are quick to prepare and cook, you can have a healthy meal every night of the week. Tinned pulses, eggs, pieces of fish, pasta, rice, liver are all quick and easy to prepare. And you can buy vegetables ready-chopped or peeled and sliced to save on labour and time. You can also double up and freeze the surplus.

But having said all that, if food is what you really enjoy, it could be that taking a bit more time to buy, cook and enjoy it is the way to go. You like your food – why not make more time for it?

Five Steps to Success

Step one

✱ *Practise mindful eating ... act holistically ... make changes*
Start mindful eating today, as outlined above. Recognise your own food triggers and try strategies to overcome them. But realise that losing weight is only partly about the actual food that you put in your mouth; it is a holistic effort involving you mind and body.

If you eat for psychological reasons you need to work on those problems alongside your poor eating patterns. Start now.

So you don't find the task ahead daunting it is best to make changes you can stick with (see 'Making Changes', above).

Step two

✱ *Become more active ... embrace life now ... don't wait*
This doesn't necessarily mean exercise, although that is certainly an important part of recovery from overeating. It means 'doing' more, especially the activities you will enjoy, rather than just 'being' – being passive, a spectator on life.

For this, I would look at what you used to enjoy as a child, teen or young adult and see if there is anything similar you can do today. Dancing, walking, visiting, talking to friends, photography, reading, writing – anything. Of all the negative emotions, it is boredom that masquerades as hunger more than any other.

Step three

✱ *Relax! ... Be happy now ... think of three good things every day*

This might seem to be the opposite of step two, but in your life there should be room both for activity and proper mind and body relaxation – OK, I hate the phrase, but it's 'me time'.

Research at Leeds University has shown that people under stress frequently prefer to choose high-fat, high-calorie foods. Relaxation techniques such as yoga, breathing control and simple 'me time' reliably reduce stress levels and are an important tool in general wellbeing. The classic picture of 'me time' is soaking in a scented bath reading or listening to music. But there are hundreds of other things that could work for you – anything that makes you laugh is brilliant for a start.

Relaxation is not simply of the body, though – it needs to be in the mind. You need to face and accept your emotions before you can truly relax. It's important to be happy *now* – not just to promise yourself you'll be happy at some time in the future (when you've lost weight, for example). At the end of every day, before you go to sleep, think of the good things about that day. And then think of three small but good things related to how you ate/drank/exercised. After you've done this for a few days, you'll be making a mental note during the day that you've achieved something that you will be able to recall at bedtime – it's a great tool for helping you to feel good about yourself.

Also try thinking about ways in which you are already benefiting from any changes you've made.

Step four

✱ *Be kind to yourself ... read your body signals ... avoid scale-hopping*

Eating has never been an exact science and you should not expect it to be one now. There will be times when you eat more than other times. This is normal, so don't beat yourself up – but you will feel better about 'lapses', if you can read your body signals.

For example, women will very often feel the need to eat more before a period. This is a natural occurrence and it is better to go with it than to try to deny it. Even better, research shows that during this phase a woman's metabolic rate rises significantly, meaning any extra calories you eat are likely to be burnt off, anyway. Those cravings are nature's way of ensuring you get enough to eat at this time – serendipity. So go with it, and eat more good, healthy food. After a period is when most women find it easiest to eat less, and that is what you should do.

You may also need to unlearn typical 'dieter's' habits. For example, long-term serial scale-hoppers should forget about the bathroom scales. Weighing is often self-defeating. The way your clothes feel and your waist measurement should tell you all you need to know.

Step five

❋ *Don't be afraid ... visualise ... be aware ... be strong*
You've read it all. You know it makes sense. But for some reason you don't apply it to yourself. For example, you have read and understood the sense of managing your own hunger/appetite and not being afraid of it, and have realised that satiety levels can be managed. Yet somehow, a little voice is telling you it isn't appropriate for you. You need to say, 'If it has worked for others, it can work for me'.

Use visualisation; it is a brilliant tool for making things happen. Visualise the long term – what your life will be like when you feel fitter, slimmer, healthier. And visualise the short term – how you're going to enjoy eating your next, healthy, meal and what size of portion you're going to give yourself, and how you're going to stop eating when you feel full up. Sportspeople use this technique – they picture themselves in the situation they will be facing (e.g. lining up for a race, feeling confident) and they picture themselves winning, several times a day. When the race happens in real life, they are more likely to get better results.

You also need to be unafraid to make your own choices. And you need to be aware. Every time you go shopping you need to remember why people are shoving food in your face, metaphorically. You need to be unafraid to be strong. This may sound like the opposite of step three. But it isn't. You can be both relaxed and strong – it's an ideal combination.

You need to want to do it and know you can do it. Because you can.

> If the strategies aren't working, change the strategies.

In conclusion, it is my hope and belief that, eventually, our food choices and decisions will be made much easier for us by a general pulling together of all the forces at play whereby good, healthy food is provided for us to eat and we are encouraged to be active in enjoyable ways – as the government admitted was the ideal way forward in its obesity report mentioned earlier.

But until that happens, most of us will have to find the right course without much in the way of high-level help. Luckily, there are millions of us in the same situation, so we must not be afraid to seek companionship, support, exercise buddies – whatever it takes. We can – and will – take control of our own bodies and our own lives.

11
The Questionnaires

In this chapter, you will learn how to put your new-found insight and knowledge to practical use through a self-help action plan for both the short and long term. No diets, no promises – just the simple application of your body IQ using questionnaires, insights and a variety of other tools.

Personal History

The first questionnaire relates to your personal history, the answers to which will lead on to my recommendations for what you should do next and will also be used in conjunction with other information in this chapter.

What is your Body Mass Index? (See p. 22 to work this out.)

- If your BMI is under 25, you may not need to lose any weight (see guidelines, p. 42). If you have a BMI of around 25, but your waist measurement is over that recommended (see p. 44) or borderline, you may simply need to do some exercise.
- If your BMI is under 22.5, but you still feel you need to lose weight, please go back and read Chapter One again and also consider contacting Beat UK (see Further Help, p. 218).
- If you do match the criteria for possibly needing to lose weight, carry on here:

Answer the following questions:

1. Have you been overweight for most of your life?

If Yes, continue here; if No, go to question 2.
Choose one of the following:

- Your BMI is up to 27 and remains steady, your waist circumference is within the guidelines for health, and you are regularly active.

Action: for your health, you may not need to do anything other than not gain any more weight, although you could also take the fitness test below, look at the type/s of activity you do and introduce more variety to ensure fitness in all three corners of the stamina/stength/flexibility triangle (see p. 165).

- Your BMI is up to 27 and remains steady, your waist circumference is within the guidelines for health, but you are inactive.
  Action: for your health, you should take the fitness test below and begin some form of regular activity (see Chapter Nine). This will also help to ensure you don't put on any more weight.
- Your BMI is over 27 and remains steady and you are regularly active.
  Action: you may need to make some difference choices in what you eat and drink or, if you are already eating healthily, then reduce portion sizes. You may also need to increase your activity levels a little or change/vary the activity you do; take the fitness test below too. Both these actions will help to reduce your weight and waist circumference.
- Your BMI is over 27 and remains steady but you are inactive.
  Action: you should take the fitness test below and begin some form of regular activity which may slowly reduce your BMI down to 27 or under and help protect your health. You should also reduce portion sizes and make some changes in your food choices, if necessary (see Chapter Five).
- Your BMI is over 27 and is regularly increasing.
  Action: you need to take the fitness test below and either begin exercise or increase exercise levels, as well as adjusting your eating habits (portions and types of food), if necessary to reduce your weight – at first to 27 or below and, if your waist circumference is still raised, until it meets the healthy criteria.

For all the above profiles, the remaining questionnaires in this chapter will be of use.

✳ Notes
If you have been overweight all your life, including childhood, this can have a profound effect on your confidence in your own ability to lose weight and get fit. You have been what you are for so long that it may seem hard to believe you can change. You need to work on getting a 'new' picture of yourself into focus, as explained in Chapter Ten.

Being slightly overweight is less of a health hazard than a lack of fitness. If you can maintain a BMI of between 25 and 27 at a steady level, you are probably doing fine.

2. Has your weight gain occurred in the past few years or less, after your having been a reasonable weight for the rest of your life?

If Yes, continue here; if No, go to question 3.

- **Has your weight gain occurred due to pregnancy?**
  This is normal.
  Action: skip the Perceptions questionnaire and go straight to Foods for You and Your Support System questionnaires (p. 213 and p. 215). Breastfeeding can help remove surplus weight. Don't be too hard on yourself in the early weeks of motherhood; but on the other hand, do try to eat healthily and get as much moderate activity as you can. Postnatal exercise is a specialist subject – ask your health visitor for advice.

- **Has your weight gain occurred due to the menopause?**
  This is normal, but not completely inevitable. Hormonal changes can affect the metabolic rate, as can the body's diminishing muscle mass during and after the menopause. Decreasing oestrogen levels can also increase the waist size.
  Action: a healthy diet, as outlined in Chapter Five, plus regular activity in all the fitness triangle corners (see p. 165) can reduce the physical effects of the menopause – take the fitness test first (p. 208). Don't attempt to slim below a reasonable weight – BMI 25–26 may be ideal to maintain bone density. Complete the remaining questionnaires in this chapter for further help.

- **Has your weight gain occurred due to illness, convalescence or enforced inactivity?**
  This is common. Illness can alter the metabolic rate – sometimes it can be speeded up, but it can also diminish, especially with prolonged bed rest and unused muscles. Some drugs can also slow the metabolism. Eating through boredom can sometimes be a factor.

Action: with your doctor's knowledge and consent, healthier snacks, small, regular meals, periods out of bed (if possible) to do gentle to moderate exercise. If health is restored, then follow action plan, depending on new weight, as explained in question 1 above.

- **Has your weight gain occurred later in life (age 60 plus)?**
  This is fairly common. The most common pattern is weight gain in our fifties and sixties, then weight reduction from the late sixties, partly due to natural shrinkage and less body fluid and partly due to diminished appetite.
  Action: drastic slimming must be avoided in later life and bone and muscle strength conserved, if at possible. This can be achieved by regular moderate weight-bearing activity, if suitable (try fitness test and see a doctor), a healthy moderate diet and reduced portions sizes to take account of your slowing metabolic rate. Continue with remaining questionnaires in this chapter.

✷ *Notes*

Weight gain due to 'life events' such as pregnancy, illness, forced inaction or prescription drugs, for example, is not *always* any easier to lose than weight which has accrued for other behavioural or psychological reasons. However, it often is. This is because a) the surplus weight was gained as a side effect of other happenings in your life, and b) the gain in these instances is not associated with all the negative feelings that often accompany weight gain (e.g. guilt, despair, depression) or the emotional reasons that are often a big factor. When the life events/happenings are removed then eating/ activity patterns may return to normal and the gained weight will be shed without much trouble. That's not to say it will go on its own. I suggest if you're wanting to lose weight after a life event, try the Your Support System questionnaire (p. 215).

3. Does your weight fluctuate on a regular basis?

If Yes, continue here; if No, go back and choose an option from question 1 or 2 which will apply to you.

- **Does your weight fluctuate because you diet to lose weight then stop dieting and put it back on?**
  This is common, especially in men and women in their thirties,

forties and fifties. You are a 'yo-yo' dieter. Getting off the yo-yo cycle isn't easy, but it can be done.

Action: most people report success if they stop trying so hard, don't follow 'diets' at all, but aim to make gradual, small changes in eating patterns that they can really stick with, combined with regular, moderate activities they enjoy, and a busy and fulfilling life. It also helps to understand the history of 'diets' – see Chapter Four, and to try the eating suggestions in Chapter Five. Chapter Ten is crucial. Continue with the remaining questionnaires in this chapter.

- **Does your weight fluctuate because sometimes you eat more, then you cut back?**
  This is fairly common. As many of us don't lead regulated lives we find that sometimes we are in 'eat' situations – e.g. a run of important dinners, an all-inclusive holiday or a working trip where healthy food choices are limited. Presto, you find you've gained half a stone – so when you have a chance, you cut back a bit.
  Action: you're dealing with normal life in the best way you can, but if you've got this far in the questionnaires, you are, nevertheless, overweight. Try to choose healthier options at regular dinners and try to get activity even when you're travelling or on holiday (especially on holiday). These lifestyle weight gains can, if you aren't careful, lead to long-term weight problems. Continue and do the remaining questionnaires to formulate the best ways for you to control your weight.

- **Does your weight fluctuate, and each time you get a bit heavier than the time before?**
  This is very common.
  Action: see yo-yo dieting in this question, above, and the information on what dieting does to you in Chapter Four.

✱ Notes

Fluctuating weight can also be linked with eating disorders such as bulimia and binge-eating syndromes, as well as with exercise addiction, depression and a range of conditions. If you think you may be in need of help for your problems reread the addictions section in Chapter Ten and I suggest you contact Beat (see Further Help, p. 218) and/or consider counselling or at least a visit to your doctor to discuss your problems.

Perceptions

This questionnaire looks at the issues that seem to be most important to you, and helps you to take the course of action that is most likely to achieve positive results.

For each of the statements below, tick the answer that most closely matches your own circumstances/beliefs.

Group 1

	DISAGREE	AGREE	STRONGLY AGREE
People never look good in clothes unless they're slim.	❑	❑	❑
I buy clothes a bit too small thinking I'll slim into them.	❑	❑	❑
I spend a lot of time worrying about my appearance.	❑	❑	❑
I often compare myself with others and think I am larger than them.	❑	❑	❑
I wonder what my friends really think of the way I look.	❑	❑	❑
I always choose clothes on the basis of whether they make me look thinner.	❑	❑	❑

Group 2

I need to lose weight for general health reasons.	❑	❑	❑
I need to lose weight for a specific health-related reason (e.g. I want to become pregnant).	❑	❑	❑
I feel that health and weight are closely related.	❑	❑	❑
I want to lose weight so I can take part in sports/activities.	❑	❑	❑
I have been told by my doctor I must lose weight.	❑	❑	❑
If it weren't for pressure on me from other people, I wouldn't bother about my weight.	❑	❑	❑

Group 3

I think I would feel much more attractive if I were slimmer.	❑	❑	❑
I would have a better relationship (with my partner) if I were slimmer.	❑	❑	❑
I would have more success in finding a partner if I were slimmer.	❑	❑	❑
I think being slimmer would improve my sex life.	❑	❑	❑

	DISAGREE	AGREE	STRONGLY AGREE

- I would feel much more confident about meeting new people if I were slim.
- I'm really fed up with having to be the life and soul of the party in order to get attention.

Group 4

- I am sure my weight holds me back from promotion at work.
- I would be much more outgoing if I lost weight.
- When I am slim there is a lot I want to do.
- I turn down opportunities because I lack self-belief.
- My weight is stopping me achieving what I want in life.
- I want to get slim once and for all, for me and no one else.

Results

Now let's see what's truly important to you. Finding important reasons to change is a significant motivation. This will be reflected in the group of questions to which you answer 'Strongly agree' the most. If there is a tie, add in your 'Agree' answers as well and choose the group that comes out on top.

✱ *Group 1*

If Group 1 contained the most 'strongly agrees' then your main motivation for changing weight is your appearance. Your self-esteem is strongly influenced by the way you look, both in the long term and on any particular day, and you feel that your friends and colleagues judge you by the way you look. Group 3 is also likely to be a high-priority group for you.

Action: as long as you are genuinely overweight, there is nothing wrong with using your appearance, and your lack of confidence in that respect, as a tool to help you lose weight. The catch is that, if you have been overweight for some long time, you are likely to have been feeling that way all the while – and thus, so far, it actually hasn't provided strong motivation for you to escape the fat trap (otherwise, you would have done something about it by now). So you need to look at a few other statements in the lists above, and see which ones resonated with you. If, for example, you strongly agreed with, 'I would feel much more confident about meeting new people if I were slim', this is an indication that you are less bothered than you think by your friends' view of you, but you'd really like to meet some new people. Write a list of five places or situations in which you'd like to meet new people. It could even be a local slimming group.

✱ Group 2

If you ticked mostly 'Strongly agree' in Group 2, health is your apparent motivation for weight loss. This can work well for some, but is also often too weak to provide the strong push that's needed, especially if it is other people telling you what you should do.

Action: a specific health target can be good – e.g. you want to get pregnant, or you've been told you can only have your operation if you lose a specific amount of weight. Another way to motivate yourself is to think of a real way that losing weight could improve your health and fitness enough to make a difference to your life in the short to mid term. For example, make a pledge to run a half marathon or a 5km (3 mile) jog in the park for charity in twelve months' time (e.g. www.raceforlife.com). That's a health reason with a goal.

✱ Group 3

If Group 3 came out on top for 'Strongly agree' answers, your main motivation is to become more sexually attractive, confident in finding or keeping a partner or in having plenty of attention and/or the ability to pick and choose. (You are also likely to have Group 1 as another high priority.) This can be a strong driving force for many people. That is why single people looking for love/sex/a partner find it easier to keep weight off than people who are happily content in a relationship. If this hasn't worked for you (i.e. you're single and available, but you are overweight), there is something you're not admitting to that is preventing you from losing weight. Perhaps your weight has become a convenient reason to stay single – are you scared? Perhaps you've been let down in love too often – a box of chocolates in front of the TV is comforting, a potential new partner a bit of a worry?

Action: maybe you simply need to be honest with yourself (it's OK, no one else is around). Give yourself some 'me time' to think it all through. What do you really want? What's holding you back? If you have a few heart-to-heart sessions with yourself like this and still can't get to the crux of it, you may need to delve a bit deeper, possibly with a little outside help. Some counselling might be useful or even a group such as Overeaters Anonymous (see Further Help, p. 218).

✱ Group 4

If you've ticked mostly 'Strongly agree' in Group 4, you want to lose weight because you feel that success and fulfilment in life are strongly linked with your weight. You tend to hold back until the day you lose weight. Most of us occasionally feel that we would have got the job if we'd paid more attention to looking smart and projecting ourselves in a favourable way. Rejection happens to us all at some point. But it is quite true, according to research, that employers tend to prefer recruiting slim people. They say, right or wrong, that fat people don't take good care of themselves and may lack discipline – two important things in the workplace. It could also be that if you go into life situations almost primed for failure (simply because your weight has lowered your self-confidence) you won't come across well.

But at the root of it all lies a confidence issue.

Action: you need to start working on improving your confidence first, before you even draw up your more moderate eating plan. That could mean not waiting until you are slim to start making your mark on life, small steps at a time. Be the first one to make a phone call. Join a group (hobby/pressure for example). Every time someone says to you, 'That's good!', or says, 'Thank you', that should increase your confidence.

You also need to start working on being in control. Look at that slice of cheesecake or bag of crisps and feel angry with it, just like I did with the packet of cigarettes (see p. 186). You're the boss.

Next ...

Depending on your results in the Perceptions questionnaire, you may need at this point to put the book down, go away – maybe even for some time – and come back when you feel you've sorted out any issues that are stopping you from having the body you want to live with. When that has happened, pick up the book again and do the test that follows:

One-minute 1–10 scale test

On a scale of 1–10, do you really, really want a better/slimmer/fitter/body? Think about it. Be honest. Put an X where you come.

1 10

On a scale of 1–10, can you really, really picture yourself as you want to be? Can you visualise yourself inside your better/slimmer/fitter body – out there, in the pool, in the changing room, in the bath?

1 10

On a scale of 1–10, do you really, really believe that you can do it (make and sustain the necessary changes) this time? Do you have the confidence? Have you read the book? Do you have the knowledge?

1 10

On a scale of 1–10, do you have an important reason (or reasons) to succeed? (If you have tried and not got there before, there needs to be a difference this time.)

1 10

If you're still hovering anywhere lower than 9 on any of the above, you're not ready; if you put your Xs in each of the tests at or near 10, you have all you need to succeed. It's time.

The Fitness Tests

From the tests below, choose the set that applies to your age group. To do the measured kilometre test you will need a pedometer (widely available and inexpensive). Whatever your result, the Further Help section will also help you source the right level and type of activity for you; and you should also read Chapter Nine.

Note: always check with your doctor before performing new exercises. This is especially important if you have any health issues, including joint pain, neck pain, back problems, high blood pressure or heart/respiratory problems. If at any time during these tests you experience pain, dizziness, faintness, palpitations or other discomfort, stop.
Always exercise when your body is warm and wear comfortable, flexible clothes.

Age under forty

✱ *Core strength*
Lie on back on mat, knees bent and feet flat on floor, arms at sides, palms down.
Concentrate on your abdominal muscles. Slowly raise your head, neck and shoulders off the floor, keeping your hands on the floor. Return. How many can you perform before you have to stop?

Repeats	Score
40 plus	4
31–40	3
21–30	2
20 or under	1

* Cardiovascular fitness

Run (or run/walk or walk, if necessary) 1 kilometre, at a pace at which you feel slightly out of breath but are in no discomfort, using a pedometer to measure distance and time. How long does it take you?

Time	Score
Under 6 minutes	4
6–7 minutes	3
7–8 minutes	2
Over 8 minutes	1

* Upper-body strength

Lie on your front on a mat with your hands beneath your shoulders, palms flat on floor. Push your body up using your hands, until your arms are straight with your lower back straight and toes flexed to support your legs. How many repeats can you do before you have to stop?

Repeats	Score
Over 25	4
20–25	3
12–19	2
11 or under	1

* Flexibility

Sit on the floor, legs together stretched out in front of you with toes pointing away from you too, and your back, including the base of your spine, against a wall. Lean forward with arms outstretched to reach towards your toes. How far can you go?

Flexibility	Score
Beyond your toes	4
Between your ankles and toes	3
Between mid-shin and ankles	2
Not as far as mid-shin	1

❋ *Your results*

Score 13–16: you are fitter than average – well done! Keep up regular exercise and activity from the stamina/strength/flexibility triangle. If you scored low in one particular area, concentrate on improving that.

Score 9–12: you are averagely fit. If you're overweight, you could increase your activity to help lose weight if you want to. Taking up a sport is a good way to keep motivated.

Score 5–8: you are not very fit. At first, concentrate on improving the area/s you scored particularly low in – for example, if you scored only one on upper-body strength, do resistance exercises to improve your arms and shoulders.

Score 4: you have a very poor fitness level. Although the good news is that you can only get better. Start with gentle, easy exercise – walking and abdominal exercises are ideal, and you will soon see results. You also need to do resistance exercise (e.g. with weights) to improve your bone density, as peak bone mass is reached in your thirties – after that it's too late.

Age forty–sixty

❋ *Core strength*

Read the instructions for previous age group, but put a small cushion under your head, if necessary. How many can you do?

Repeats	Score
Over 30	4
21–30	3
11–20	2
10 or under	1

❋ *Cardiovascular fitness*

Jog or jog/run or briskly walk, at a pace at which you feel slightly out of breath, but are in no discomfort, for 1 kilometre, using a pedometer to measure distance and time. How long does it take you?

Time	Score
Under 7 minutes	4
7–8 minutes	3
8–9 minutes	2
Over 9 minutes	1

✳ Upper-body strength

Kneel on the floor on all fours with your knees approximately 15cm (6in) back from your hips (so your upper legs are not quite at right angles to floor), palms flat on the floor, below your shoulders. Dip down to the floor, bending your arms and keeping your palms still. Raise up again. How many of these moves can you do before you have to stop?

Repeats	Score
Over 25	4
20–25	3
12–19	2
11 or under	1

✳ Flexibility

Follow the instructions for the previous group. How far can you go?

Flexibility	Score
To the base of your toes or beyond	4
Between your ankles and toes	3
Between mid-shin and ankles	2
To upper shin or less	1

✳ Your results

Score 13–16: you have an excellent all-round fitness level for your age. If you continue to exercise regularly you can keep a high percentage of your current fitness into older age, and help prevent 'middle-age spread'. If you scored lower on one particular test, pay more attention to that area of the fitness triangle.

Score 9–12: you have average fitness for your age. This is good, but you could perhaps consider doing more, as without exercise, lean tissue (muscle) is lost during mid life, and for women, after the menopause, resistance exercise helps prevent bone loss.

Score 5–8: you are below average fitness for your age. You've probably fallen into the trap of tailing off your activity as you've got older. It's certainly not too late to increase this once more though – all research shows you can regain most, if not all, of the fitness you may have had when younger. Chapter Nine should provide plenty of ideas.

Score 4: you have a poor level of fitness for your age, but don't worry – if you want to get fitter, you definitely can, and doing so will make a real difference if you need to lose weight or find it hard to maintain a reasonable weight. The good news is that very unfit people make quick progress – as long as you start with easy, gentle sessions. And once you're fit, you don't have to do huge amounts to stay that way.

Age over sixty

* Core strength
Follow the instructions for the previous group, but put a small cushion under your head. How many can you do?

Repeats	Score
Over 20	4
11–20	3
5–10	2
4 or under	1

* Cardiovascular fitness
Walk for 1 kilometre at as fast a pace as you can comfortably go without feeling breathless or being unable to talk.

Time	Score
Under 10 minutes	4
10–11 minutes	3
11–12 minutes	2
Over 12 minutes	1

* Flexibility
Follow the instructions for the previous group. How far can you go?

Flexibility	Score
To your feet	4
To your ankles	3
To mid-shin	2
To knees or less	1

* Your results
Score 9–12: congratulations – you are above average fitness for your age! The activity that you regularly get is helping you to maintain your muscle and bone, as well as providing many other benefits which will see you into a

healthy old age. There's no reason why you can't continue to exercise whatever your age and, as your metabolic rate slows down as you age, it will also help you keep slim.

Score 5–8: you have average fitness for your age, so you're not doing badly. But go back and see which area you scored least well in, and try to include more exercise on a regular basis to improve that area. For example, if you did poorly on the walking test, try to improve your stamina levels. It's also important to do regular flexibility exercise to maintain supple joints and help prevent aches and pains.

Score under 5: you have below average fitness for your age, so it's important to try to build some more activity into your life on a regular basis; most of us can do something. You could begin with a short daily walk, or even stair-climbing or a DVD workout, especially designed for your age group.

Foods For You

So far, food has hardly been mentioned in this chapter. Yet food (and drink, maybe) is a big issue. What you eat has to fit in well with your life, and you need to enjoy it, or no amount of motivation will work. So let's just take a small detour, and revisit a few of the ways in which you can eat well and feel happy, whatever your lifestyle and preferences.

From the statements below, simply choose the one that most closely matches your needs, then read all the lovely foods that will fit in with your life.

- **I need quick, easy food that fits in with my fast-paced lifestyle.**
  Carbs: wholegrain bread, pasta, two-minute brown basmati rice, bulgur wheat, wholegrain breakfast cereals.
  Protein: fish fillets, smoked salmon, chicken breasts, steaks, lean burgers, two-minute microwave lentils, omelette/scrambled eggs, low- to medium-fat cheese, yogurt, milk, nuts, seeds.
  Fat: salmon fillets, mackerel fillets, nuts, seeds, salad oils.
  Vegetables: bagged salads, ready-prepared vegetables, bean sprouts, frozen peas, beans, broccoli, carrots.
  Fruit: apples, pears, plums, bananas, grapes, blueberries, raspberries.

- **I need low-cost food as I'm on a tight budget.**
  Carbs: wholegrain bread (try making your own using 'just add

water' bread flour), wholewheat pasta, brown basmati rice, bulgur wheat, wholegrain breakfast cereals, potatoes.
Protein: eggs, lean burgers, lean beef, turkey, lamb or pork mince, lentils/lentil soup, chick peas, kidney beans, baked beans, milk, yogurt.
Fat: fresh/frozen mackerel, herring fillets, sardines, canned mackerel, sardines, rapeseed oil, groundnut oil.
Vegetables: many vegetables in season – buy and freeze or buy in bulk and share with neighbours; frozen vegetables – look out for offers and buy when cheap.
Fruit: choose fruits in season and, again, buy and freeze or share.

- **I need comforting, tasty family food that everyone will enjoy.**
  Carbs: bread, pittas, rolls, bagels, baps, malt loaf, hot cross buns, teacakes, rice, couscous, unsweetened breakfast cereals, potatoes, oven chips, pasta bakes, wholewheat pancakes.
  Protein: egg frittata or omelettes, baked fish, fish pie, lean burgers, bean burgers, lentil soup, baked beans, lean minced beef/pork/ turkey/chicken, milk, yogurt, fromage frais, moderate-fat cheeses, lean roast meat, lean ham.
  Fat: salmon burgers, mackerel pâté, nuts, seeds, salad oils.
  Vegetables: peas, carrots, beans, tomatoes, onions, peppers, courgettes, stir-fried shredded cabbage, any vegetables made into soup or pasta sauce.
  Fruit: fruit crumbles made with oat and wholemeal topping, baked apples, pears poached in juice, dried fruit compote with chopped nuts, baked bananas, pineapple and banana stir-fried in butter and orange juice.

This detour should hopefully have served as a reminder that eating well means just that – eating well, not depriving yourself or having to alter your lifestyle completely. Whoever you are, whatever you do, there's good food out there that will help you.

Your Support System

When we set out to achieve something – no matter how strong our motivation and determination – it always helps to have a support system in place. Depending on your personality type and your own 'mind games' (which may be in place because of your weight issues themselves), the type of support you go for can be different. Several different 'types' are described below, along with the kind of support that will be most useful for them, in terms of both diet and activity. Choose the type that matches most closely the way you are at present.

- **I am – or used to be – a 'people person' – I feel happy as part of a team, it brings out the best in me.**
  Diet: you will do well in a group – maybe a group of colleagues or neighbours – who all have similar weight-loss goals. You could set targets, make comparisons and set yourselves challenges.
  Activity: again, the same group – or a different one – could organise activities together, from a walk or jog in the park to visits to the leisure centre or even active holidays.

- **I enjoy being led/helped and work best when given instruction.**
  Diet: you're an ideal candidate for a local slimming club, where you'll get personal advice and attention.
  Activity: you may do well at the gym or an exercise class.

- **I am used to being a leader rather than a follower.**
  Diet: if you're used to being boss, you won't take kindly to a slimming group or even a programme designed for you online. You need freeform help – set your own targets and goals and stick to them by finding someone (or more than one person) you would let down if you don't achieve. This might be giving money to charity for every pound lost, for example.
  Activity: you could start up your own group (it's not hard to find willing participants in your area, either by going to one of the many social networking sites online or advertising on your local town website) and designate yourself chairperson, so you can decide what the group does. Various official websites provide information on exercise and activity ideas and, importantly, health and safety considerations (see Further Help, p. 218).

- **I tend to be a loner and work best by myself, making my own decisions.**

  Diet: your support needs to be via self-feedback. Keep a daily food diary with comments alongside on how you felt about what you ate, notes to yourself about days or times you felt less positive, more positive and so on. Although I don't normally recommend regular weighing, a fortnightly (NOT more frequent) weighing session may be a good idea to keep track of pounds lost. And regularly measuring your waist will keep you motivated should weight loss be low.

  Activity: similarly, keep an exercise diary. Improving on your results week on week is a very strong motivation. If you have room, get some pieces of home exercise equipment that you fancy, say, a bike which records time, distance, pace, calories burnt, difficulty and so on. Consider getting a dog or maybe dog-walking for neighbours.

- **I think I do need support, but I prefer to trust close family or one or two friends.**

  Diet: family can be brilliant support – or they can be top notch saboteurs. If your family or friends also want to shape up, they could be just the people you need around you – you can encourage each other. But even if they don't, you could still get one of them to be your designated home tutor – they just need to be willing to weigh/measure you once a fortnight or so and offer words of encouragement – hopefully not admonishment. But if your family are not supportive of your weight-loss efforts, and there is no one else you can trust, you might find an online designated chat room (e.g. at Weight Loss Resources, Netmums or iVillage) helpful. You can say what you like, have a rant (and get some good advice sometimes) without fear of exposing yourself.

  Activity: rope in the family or a friend for regular walks, cycle rides, sessions in the garden or park with a bat and ball – making things fun will help keep them interested. There's no need to mention that you're doing it for your figure. In winter, consider persuading your best friend to join a dance class with you; from line dancing to jazz – it's all good.

- **It makes me feel good to help others, to 'put something back'.**
  Diet: you need to turn your weight-loss campaign into a good cause – do it for charity. Raise sponsorship to slim.
  Activity: you can do sponsored walks, runs or events (e.g. for The Children's Trust or the British Heart Foundation) and/or work activity into a help task – for example, walking around your neighbourhood selling raffle tickets or offering your services to help train the local girls' (or boys') football team.

- **I'm a homebody – whatever help I get, it needs to be at home.**
  Diet: there are several ways you can do this – enlist family or flatmates to keep an eye on your progress (see above), or online/postal/telephone help. Various slimming clubs and organisations will give you this help. You can take the bits you want and leave the rest (see Chapter Eight).
  Activity: an exercise/dance DVD or Wii Fit in your sitting room would be perfect. Or, if you have room, any types of home exercise equipment (for ideas, see p. 177).

So you've reached this far. Well done. I hope and believe that you now have all the information and motivation you need to take back your own body from everyone who has been trying to snatch it away from you and call it their own.

Your body IS yours – yours to look after. It is your responsibility – but that's no bad thing. And your body is yours to celebrate. It should be your pleasure too – as should good food and good exercise.

I wrote this book because I was so exasperated with the conspiracy to keep you in permanent angst. I do think there is a change in the air – and I hope that I've helped to let you see the bigger picture and smooth and hurry the changes along.

Now go and enjoy your life, your body, your food – and look and feel better than you ever did before.

Further Help

Chapter One

* *Beat*
Tel: 0845 634 1414
Email:help@b-eat.co.uk
www.b-eat.co.uk
Formerly Eating Disorders Association.
Help and information for eating disorder
sufferers and their families.

* *National Centre for Eating Disorders*
Tel: 0845 838 2040
Email: via link on website
www.eating-disorders.org.uk
Help and advice about eating disorders
and network of trained therapists.

* *Body Gossip*
Email: info@bodygossip.org
www.bodygossip.org
Friendly pro-active site for people with
body image problems.

* *You is for Unique: Women's Feelings
About Body Image and Self-esteem*
Julia Hague (Grosvenor House
Publishing, 2009)
Women discuss their true feelings about
their looks and body issues.

Chapter Two

* *Change for Life*
Tel: 0300 123 4567
www.nhs.uk/change4life

NHS website for families wanting to live
a healthier, more balanced lifestyle.

* *National Obesity Forum*
Tel: 0115 846 2109
Email: info@nof.uk.com
www.nationalobesityforum.org.uk
Forum for obesity professionals but with
excellent help pages for individuals and
families.

* *Overeaters Anonymous*
Tel: 07000 784985
Email: general@oagb.org.uk or
oagbnsb@hotmail.com
www.oagb.org.uk
Run on similar lines to AA – regular first-
name-only group sessions.

* *Alcoholics Anonymous*
Tel: 0845 769 7555
Email: help@alcoholics-
anonymous.org.uk
www.alcoholics-anonymous.org.uk
Regular meetings – first-name-only
basis – for people with alcohol
problems.

Chapter Three

* *The Green Food Bible*
Judith Wills (Eden Project Books, 2008)
Implications of how and what we eat on
the future of the planet.

* US National Heart, Lung, and Blood Institute
www.nhlbisupport.com/bmi
Calculate your BMI easily online and assess your risk and take an interesting look at the US view of our obesity and health problems.

* British Heart Foundation
Tel: 0300 330 3311 (heart helpline)
Email: internet@bhf.org.uk
www.bhf.org.uk
Information on every aspect of heart disease prevention including diet and lifestyle advice.

* Diabetes UK
Tel: 020 7424 1000
Email: info@diabetes.org.uk
www.diabetes.org.uk
Largest UK diabetes charity – information and help.

Chapter Four

* Food Standards Agency/Eat Well
Tel: 020 7276 8829
Email: helpline@foodstandards. gsi.gov.uk
www.eatwell.gov.uk
Information and advice on healthy eating for individuals.

* Dr Robert Hill
Consultant Clinical Psychologist in Addictions,
South London and Maudsley NHS Foundation Trust.
Email: Drrghill@ntlworld.com
One of the UK's leading specialists in addictions of all kinds.

* International Journal of Obesity
Tel: 020 7833 4000
www.nature.com
Up-to-date publication of research into obesity and its causes.

Chapter Six

* Medical Research Council
Tel: 020 7636 5422
Email: corporate@headoffice.mrc.ac.uk
www.mrc.ac.uk
Publicly funded organisation for research into improving health.

* Glycaemic Index Database
www.glycemicindex.com
The official website for the Glycaemic Index and GI database, recommended by Diabetes UK.

* Weight Loss Resources
Tel: 01733 345592
Email: helpteam@weightlossresources. co.uk
www.weightlossresources.co.uk
Excellent and trustworthy online help for all things weight related.

* National Institutes of Health
Tel: 001 301-496-4000
Email: NIHinfo@od.nih.gov
http://health.nih.gov
US national medical research agency with a consumer information section on its website.

Chapter Eight

* *British Association of Aesthetic Plastic Surgeons*
Tel: 020 7405 2234
Email: info@baaps.org.uk
www.baaps.org.uk
Not a regulatory body but site contains useful information.

* *Advertising Standards Authority*
Tel: 020 7492 2222
Email: enquiries@asa.org.uk
www.asa.org.uk
Handles complaints about adverts in the UK.

Chapter Nine

* *World Health Organisation*
Tel: 00 41 22 791 21 11
Email: info@who.int
www.who.int
Includes obesity and activity pages with data and information.

* *Fitness Industry Association*
Tel: 020 7420 8560
www.fia.org.uk
Helps you find gym/class/club facilities online and runs the MoreActive4Life campaign to help encourage families to exercise.

* *British Association of Sports and Exercise Sciences*
Tel: 0113 8126162
Email: Use form on website
www.bases.org.uk
Interesting background about the science and physiology of exercise.

* *Live Well*
www.nhs.uk/LiveWell/Fitness
Government site with good motivational fitness pages and info including comprehensive search engine to find activities in your area.

* *Active Places*
www.activeplaces.co.uk
Fast, easy-to-use facility for finding any activity near you – but England only.

* *Bubl Information Service*
http://bubl.ac.uk/uk/bubluksport.htm
Online listing for all sporting organisations in the UK.

* *UK Sport*
Tel: 020 7211 5100
Email: info@uksport.gov.uk
www.uksport.gov.uk
The UK's governing body for sport.

* *Gymophobics*
Tel: 01785 227273
Email: enquiries@gymophobics.co.uk
www.gymophobics.co.uk
Female-only chain of exercise clubs.

* *Lizzie Webb/Creativity in Sport*
Email: info@creativityinsport.com
www.creativityinsport.com
Inspiration from the fitness guru.

* *AudioFuel*
Email: contact@audiofuel.co.uk
www.audiofuel.co.uk
Website where you can download music and audio coaching to listen to while running.

* *Run to the Beat*
Tel: 020 8233 5900
www.runtothebeat.co.uk
Half-marathon run in London with
website providing lots of running
information, including training tips
and nutrition.

* *Walks with Buggies*
Email: via link on website
www.walkswithbuggies.com
Provides information on walks suitable
for those with buggies and young
children.

* *Virtual Gym*
Email: info@virtualgym.tv
www.virtualgym.tv
Subscription-based website offering
downloadable workout sessions.

* *The Green Gym*
Tel: 01302 388 883
Email: information@btcv.org.uk
www2.btcv.org.uk
Volunteer for outdoor work – improve
health and environment.

Chapter Ten

* *The Wild Life: A Year of Living on
Wild Food*
John Lewis Stempel (Doubleday & Co
inc., 2009).
Fascinating insight into eating to
survive, and how it changes attitudes
to food.

* *Applied Cognitive and Behavioural
Approaches to the Treatment of Addiction:
A Practical Treatment Guide*
Mitcheson, L., Maslin. J., Meynon, T.,
Morrison, T., Hill, R.G., & Wanigaratne,
S. (Wiley Blackwell, 2009).
A professional analysis of how CBT can
help cure addictions.

* *Excessive Appetites: A Psychological
View of Addictions*
Jim Oford (John Wiley and Sons, 2001).
Book covering all addictions, including
eating and alcohol.

* *The End of Overeating: Taking Control
of the Insatiable American Appetite*
Dr David Kessler (Rodale Press, 2009).
An interesting insight into why
populations eat too much.

* *Cognitive Behavioural Therapy (CBT)*
British Association for Behavioural and
Cognitive Psychotherapies
Tel: 0161 797 4484
Email: babcp@babcp.com
www.babcp.com
Find a therapist on site – also links to
other useful sources.

* *Hypnosis*
British Society of Clinical Hypnosis
Tel: 01262 403103
Email: sec@bsch.org.uk
www.bsch.org.uk
Learn more about hynotherapy and find
a practitioner.

Index